Emergency Medical Services Systems

HEALTH AFFAIRS INFORMATION GUIDE SERIES

Series Editor: Winifred Sewell, Health Science Information Consultant, currently associated with the University of Maryland and the National Health Planning Information Center

Also in this series:

BIOETHICS—*Edited by Doris Goldstein**

CROSS-NATIONAL STUDY OF HEALTH SYSTEMS: CONCEPTS, METHODS, AND DATA SOURCES—*Edited by Ray H. Elling*

CROSS-NATIONAL STUDY OF HEALTH SYSTEMS: COUNTRIES, WORLD REGIONS, AND SPECIAL PROBLEMS—*Edited by Ray H. Elling*

HEALTH CARE ADMINISTRATION—*Edited by Dwight A. Morris and Lynne Darby Morris*

HEALTH CARE COSTS AND FINANCING—*Edited by Rita Keintz*

HEALTH MAINTENANCE THROUGH FOOD AND NUTRITION—*Edited by Helen D. Ullrich*

HEALTH STATISTICS—*Edited by Frieda O. Weise*

HUMAN ECOLOGY—*Edited by Frederick Sargent II**

THE PROFESSIONAL AND SCIENTIFIC LITERATURE ON PATIENT EDUCATION—*Edited by Lawrence W. Green and Connie Cavanaugh Kansler*

*in preparation

The above series is part of the
GALE INFORMATION GUIDE LIBRARY

The Library consists of a number of separate series of guides covering major areas in the social sciences, humanities, and current affairs.

General Editor: Paul Wasserman, Professor and former Dean, School of Library and Information Services, University of Maryland

Managing Editor: Denise Allard Adzigian, Gale Research Company

Emergency Medical Services Systems

A GUIDE TO INFORMATION SOURCES

Volume 9 in the Health Affairs Information Guide Series

Carlos Fernández-Caballero

former Director
National Emergency Medical Services
Information Clearinghouse
University of Pennsylvania

with

Marianne Fernández-Caballero

Librarian
Samuel Paley Library
Temple University
Philadelphia

Gale Research Company
Book Tower, Detroit, Michigan 48226

Library of Congress Cataloging in Publication Data

Fernández-Caballero, Carlos.
   Emergency medical services systems.

   (Health affairs information guide series ; v. 9)
(Gale information guide library)
   Includes indexes.
   1. Emergency medical services—Bibliography.
2. Emergency medical services—United States—
Bibliography. 3. Emergency medical services—
Information services—United States—Directories.
4. Emergency medical services—United States—
Societies, etc.—Directories. I. Fernández-
Caballero, Marianne. II. Title. III. Series.
Z6675.E45F47   [RA645.5]   016.616′025   81-13295
ISBN 0-8103-1503-3   AACR2

Copyright © 1981 by
Carlos Fernández-Caballero and Marianne Fernández-Caballero

No part of this book may be reproduced in any form without permission in writing from the publisher, except by a reviewer who wishes to quote brief passages or entries in connection with a review written for inclusion in a magazine or newspaper. Manufactured in the United States of America.

VITAE

Carlos Fernández-Caballero holds a diploma in librarianship from the National University of Cordoba, Argentina, and a master of science from Syracuse University, School of Library Science. He is currently working on his Ph.D. dissertation at the University of Pennsylvania.

Carlos Fernández-Caballero was director of the library at the Faculty of Sciences, University of Cuyo, Argentina; chief librarian, Binational Center, Asuncion, Paraguay; librarian, Institute of Sciences of the National University of Asuncion; cataloger, the Library of Congress, Washington, D.C.; supervisor of technical services, Prince William County Public Library System, Manassas, Virginia; professor of library science at the School of Librarians, National University of Asuncion; and director of the University of Pennsylvania, National Emergency Medical Services Information Clearinghouse (NEMSIC).

Marianne Fernández-Caballero received a bachelor of arts degree with final honors in 1968 from Mary Washington College, Fredericksburg, Virginia, and graduated from Drexel University, Philadelphia, in 1975 with a master of science in library science degree and special training in medical librarianship and bibliography. While studying at Drexel, she was employed by the Library of the College of Physicians of Philadelphia. Marianne Fernández-Caballero, who has also worked as a cataloger at the Library of Congress, is presently a cataloger at the Samuel Paley Library of Temple University in Philadelphia.

CONTENTS

Foreword	ix
Introduction	xiii
Abbreviations Used in the Text	xv

Chapter 1. Emergency Medical Services Systems:
Overview	1
A. Organization	1
B. Funding	2
EMS Act Funded Programs	3
C. Legislation	4

Chapter 2. Sources	5
A. Information Centers	5
B. Bibliographies	6
C. Computerized Data Base	12
D. Periodicals	12
Journals	13
Newsletters	16
E. Audiovisual Aids	24

Chapter 3. Emergency Medical Services
Organizations	27
A. Organizations—Direct Involvement With EMS	27
B. Organizations—Peripheral Involvement With EMS	29
C. Governmental and Official (or Semiofficial Agencies)	29

Chapter 4. Literature	31
A. Manpower and Training	31
B. Communications	45
C. Transportation	52
General	53
Ambulances	57
Mobile Coronary Care Units (MCCU)	69
Air Transportation	73
D. Facilities	79
Categorization	79
Utilization	89
E. Critical Care Units	104
Trauma	104
Burn Care	108

Contents

	Spinal Cord Injury	111
	Poisoning	112
	Acute Cardiac Care	114
	High Risk Infant	114
	Behavioral Emergencies	117
	Public Safety Agencies	119
	Consumer Participation	120
F.	Accessibility to Care	121
G.	Coordinated Patient Record Keeping	122
H.	Public Information and Education	127
I.	Review and Evaluation	129
J.	Disaster Plan--Mutual Aid	143

Appendix. Regional Consultants and State Coordinators for Emergency Medical Services ... 153

Author Index ... 159
Title Index ... 167
Subject Index ... 173

FOREWORD

Interest in health and the resources and activities that make it possible is not new. However, the concepts of health as a national resource and as a human right have emerged in the recent past. Legislation during the last two decades has led from these concepts to a complex system with some unsurprising growing pains.

Many people have come into the field, bringing a multiplicity of backgrounds to supplement the traditional health sciences. In addition, today's laymen must make decisions on health care at all levels--from voting for or against legislators who will shape health laws, through serving on local health planning boards, to becoming participants in informed decisions on their own health care. The new recruits and the laymen have in common the need for all kinds of information on social, business, legal, ethical, and other aspects of medicine.

Much of this information has previously been unavailable and not readily understandable to the new audiences. Attempts to satisfy the need have resulted in burgeoning publications on a variety of subjects, ranging from the broad to the specific. These new publications are in many forms, from carefully edited, important texts to poorly conceived and executed technical reports, with a vast array in between. There are journals, newsletters, association and university guidebooks and models, statistical reports, and audiovisuals--all with varying quality and format.

Several problems have resulted. In the first place, there has not yet emerged a major bibliographic resource, such as the National Library of Medicine and Excerpta Medica provide for the clinical and research aspects of medicine. Those who have access to MEDLINE services have recently been enabled to find at least a part of the pertinent current periodical references through the new data base, health planning and administration, or FILE HEALTH. A second problem is that some of the novices in the field are not accustomed to using published literature in any form, let alone the complex of primary, secondary, and tertiary publications with which their counterparts in clinical medicine and research have become familiar.

It is the purpose of the Health Affairs Series in the Gale Information Guide Library to provide guides for participants in the complex health care system to information on the system itself--on the process of the delivery of health care. We are concerned with the management of the system and with how

Foreword

researchers, educators, and practitioners assure the best health possible to each individual. We are not concerned with the content of the information with which the researcher, educator, or practitioner deals, but rather with his mode of functioning in a real world of people with different racial, ethnic, sexual, financial, and geographic backgrounds. For example, we are not interested in how a surgical procedure is carried out, but we are concerned with its availability to those who need it. If one understands the social sciences broadly, then the Health Affairs Series deals with the social aspects of medicine.

Due to time constraints for completing the series, some of our original plans have been changed. However, we hope the volumes remaining will provide a useful picture of some of the areas where the need is greatest. Individual volumes cover: Health Statistics, Human Ecology, Health Maintenance Through Food and Nutrition, The Professional and Scientific Literature of Patient Education, Cross-National Study of Health Systems, Health Care Costs and Financing, Health Care Administration, Bioethics.

The user may ask, "Why another bibliography when there are already so many?" We agree, but the Health Affairs Guides are much more than bibliographies. All contain a careful selection of materials for the intended audience, an evaluation of these materials in annotations and introductory paragraphs, and directions for finding further information. There are lists of many sources of information, such as information centers, schools, publishers, and audiovisuals. The journals which one should read regularly to keep up with the field are mentioned and annotated. In short, the reader will find specific resources for the present, and, for the future, methods of finding new sources as they are developed.

Because all of the social sciences dealing with health affairs are interrelated, it is both impossible and undesirable to prescribe strict limits for each individual volume, excluding from one anything included in another. Instead, each volume of the series is complete for the individual who is interested in only one specific subject. At the same time, other volumes serve as excellent supplements when the user wishes to go into related topics in greater depth. The series editor takes responsibility for the general organization and coverage of the series, but has left to the judgment of the volume editors decisions on individual items to be included or excluded. The series should be helpful to users not only for what they are able to find in the individual volumes, but for how it has been sifted to exclude those materials that would send them down blind alleys.

We hope that our audience for the series will consist of newcomers to the fields involved, as well as researchers and practitioners who have worked with health affairs in the past but need to renew their familiarity with resources in some aspect of their major current interests. We hope especially that the guides will be useful in the education of students who have chosen one or more of the fields covered for their future careers. And finally, we have tried to make the volumes simple and direct enough that they will provide the informed layperson with access to the information resources needed to make decisions about future procedures and policies in assurance of the best match between national resources and the health care of the nation.

Foreword

Carlos Fernández-Caballero has had much experience in the practicalities of providing information on emergency medical services to a variety of audiences. This background, together with his bibliographic expertise, has enabled him to prepare a volume which should be useful to those concerned with any aspect of the delivery of emergency health care.

Winifred Sewell, Series Editor
Cabin John, Maryland

INTRODUCTION

Accidental death and disability were once considered the "neglected disease of modern society" (1966). Many changes have altered the environment of emergency medical services (EMS) since that date. One landmark was the National Highway Safety Act of 1966, Standard 11. Following this act, through the late sixties and early seventies, federal, state and local officials, medical and other health practitioners, and even the general public became more aware of EMS. As a result, health professionals began to organize to improve emergency medical care. Physicians joined together to establish professional associations concerned with EMS, including the American College of Emergency Physicians (ACEP), the University Association for Emergency Medical Services, the American Trauma Society, and the Society for Critical Care Medicine. Nurses organized to form the Emergency Department Nurses Association (EDNA), and EMTs were banded together by the National Registry of Emergency Medical Technicians.

This increased awareness and concern was reflected in the establishment of many periodicals devoted to EMS. The Illinois Department of Health, Bureau of Emergency Medical Services and Highway Safety began to publish Trauma Center Newsletter in November 1971. In 1972 ACEP began issuing the Journal of the American College of Emergency Physicians (JACEP); EDNA initiated the publication of the Journal of Emergency Nursing (JEN) in 1975; the American Medical Association started to publish Emergency Medicine Today; the Society of Critical Care Medicine initiated the publication of Critical Care Medicine; and the Emergency Care Information Center began to print Medical 911 and EMS Communicator. All this was followed by many more publications sponsored by different groups.

The developing interest in EMS was also reflected in book publishing. Among the major works were Neil L. Chayet's Legal Implications of Emergency Care (1969), John W. Camden's Emergency Medical Services (1972), and John H. Noble's Emergency Medical Services (1973). Many training manuals were also published.

Federal agencies, such as the Rescue and Emergency Medical Services Division of the National Highway Safety Administration (Department of Transportation) and the Division of Emergency Medical Services, Department of Health and Human Services, sponsored many reports, articles, and standards related to EMS, in addition to several audiovisual aids. Many private foundations and professional societies added to this printed and audiovisual material through their grants for research and public education.

Introduction

In November 1973, PL 93-154, the Emergency Medical Services Systems Act, gave additional impetus to research and publications about EMS; it was amended in 1976 (PL 94-573) and 1979 (PL 96-142). A major commitment of funds to EMS by the Robert Wood Johnson Foundation further stimulated this trend. As a result of all these developments, there is no lack of information about EMS.

This guide is based on and enlarges upon <u>Survey of EMS Resources and Literature</u>,[1] published originally in February 1975, in collaboration with S.A. Otterbein. Now we are facing the responsibility of issuing this selected compilation of EMS data which is intended to serve as a key to widely dispersed basic information and to the identification of sources for additional research. This guide is designed for EMS administrators, public service officers, students of EMS, and people of all levels of interest in EMS.

We have chosen the items included in this guide based on our five years' experience with the management of emergency medical services information. Some of the criteria utilized in selection are: (1) qualifications expertise of the author, (2) importance of the subject covered, (3) presence in the work of useful data, and (4) geographical distribution.

The arrangement is in accordance with the fifteen components of an EMS System recommended by the EMS Act of 1976. Some components have been combined because, at times, it is difficult to classify an item in only one component because its subject matter crosses component boundaries, e.g., manpower and education. Some of the components have few items because they have not yet attracted the attention of authors, such as public safety agencies, and accessibility to care. The items are sequentially numbered to facilitate indexing. They are arranged in alphabetical order in each division.

Code numbers or identification numbers have been included for documents distributed by NTIS to assist in ordering materials. We tried to deliver the most complete data possible on all items, but sometimes found information not available, for example, names of publishers, original dates of publication for periodicals, and phone numbers for organizations.

We would like to thank Scott A. Otterbein, C. Gene Cayten, and our editor, Ms. Winifred Sewell, for all the good advice and collaboration received.

---

1. Philadelphia, National Emergency Medical Services Information Clearinghouse, University of Pennsylvania, February 1975. 43 p. 3d ed., May 1976. 59 p.

ABBREVIATIONS USED IN THE TEXT

AAAM	American Association for Automotive Medicine
AAOS	American Academy of Orthopaedic Surgeons
ACEP	American College of Emergency Physicians
ACLS	Advanced Cardiac Life Support
ACS	American College of Surgeons
AMES	Air Medical Evacuation System
BLS	Basic Life Support
CCU	Coronary Care Unit
CPR	cardiopulmonary resuscitation
DHEW	Department of Health, Education and Welfare
DOT	Department of Transportation
ECG	electrocardiogram
ED	emergency department
EDNA	Emergency Department Nurses Association
EKG	electrocardiogram
EMS	emergency medical services
EMSIC	Emergency Medical Services Information Center
EMSS	emergency medical services system
EMT	emergency medical technician
EMT-A	emergency medical technician-ambulance
EMT-P	emergency medical technician-paramedic
ER	emergency room
ERIC	Educational Resources Information Clearinghouse
IAATM	International Association for Accident and Traffic Medicine
ICU	intensive care unit
JACEP	Journal of the American College of Emergency Physicians
JAMA	Journal of the American Medical Association
JEN	Journal of Emergency Nursing
MAST	Military Assistance to Safety and Traffic

Abbreviations

MCCU	mobile coronary care unit
MICU	mobile intensive care unit
MIENS	Maryland Institute of Emergency Medical Services
NASAR	National Association of Search and Rescue
NATO	North Atlantic Treaty Organization
NEMSIC	National Emergency Medical Services Information Clearinghouse
NTIS	National Technical Information Service
OR	operation room
PHS	Public Health Service
SCI	spinal cord injury

Chapter 1
EMERGENCY MEDICAL SERVICES SYSTEMS: OVERVIEW

Emergency Medical Services Systems (EMSS) (PL 93-154) is understood as:
a system which provides for the arrangement of personnel, facilities, and equipment for the effective and coordinated delivery in an appropriate geographical area of health care services under emergency conditions, occurring either as a result of the patient's condition or of a natural disaster or similar situation, and which is administered by a public or nonprofit private entity which has the authority and the resources to provide effective administration of the system.

Although this definition mentions "under emergency" conditions, the fact is that emergency departments are utilized by thousands of citizens who do not have a "personal" physician, clogging in this manner the ED with routine nonemergency cases that better belong with the family physician or the walk-in clinic.

As a consequence of the situation explained above, the EMSS--through the emergency department--became a point of entrance for many patients to the general health (medical) system. Otherwise that would not happen because of the lack of the natural connection to the "system," a family, or personal physician. This also points up the fact that the EMSS is but a part of the general health care organization.

A. ORGANIZATION

An EMSS is based on a State Lead Agency. This body ought to have among other aspects: (1) coordination capability, at all levels and functions of the system; (2) technical and medical know-how to provide the necessary assistance to their members; and (3) ability to work with professional societies and all other institutions with primary or secondary interest in EMS.

The EMSS Act, 1973, describes the fifteen necessary components of an EMSS. They are: (1) provision of manpower (personnel); (2) (adequate) training of personnel; (3) communications; (4) transportation; (5) facilities; (6) critical care units; (7) use of (cooperation with all) public safety agencies; (8) consumer participation; (9) accessibility (for everybody) to care; (10) patient transfer; (11) coordinated patient record keeping; (12) public (consumer) information and education; (13) review and evaluation; (14) disaster plan; and (15) mutual aid (agreement and cooperation). The 1973 EMSS Act gives enough

Overview

elbow room in such matters as: planning, organization, management, financial sources, and other aspects not specifically contemplated in the law.

One aspect in which the legislation is strict is the so-called "medical control and accountability." This point was hotly argued by nonphysician administrators who believe the law empowers physicians with decision-making powers in areas where they do not have expertise, such as planning. It is considered that most average physicians are not capable of functioning properly in an emergency situation. On this matter, the <u>EMSS Guidelines</u> state:

> A physician who is acceptable to the medical community as well as knowledgeable in the planning and implementation of the EMS System is essential at both the State lead agency level and the regional EMS level. This administrative position assures medical soundness and appropriateness of all aspects of the program.
> In each situation, the medical director must be responsible for the concept system's design and overall supervision of the EMS medical program (p. 24).

B. FUNDING

The EMSS development has been funded primarily by the federal government, starting with the National Highway Safety Act of 1966, which provided funds for ambulances, communications, training, and statewide programs. This act led to the systematized organization at all levels of EMS.

Private funding was provided by the Robert Wood Johnson Foundation in 1973: $15 million, for forty-four EMS projects around the country. This was the largest amount of private funds ever allocated to emergency medical services.

The great federal funding push came from the Emergency Medical Services Systems Act of 1973 (PL 93-154, November 16, 1973), amended by PL 94-573, October 21, 1976, and by PL 96-142, December 12, 1979. This law provided federal monies for the establishment of emergency care programs. The main grants are provided under: Section 1202, Grants and Contracts for Feasibility Studies and Planning; Section 1203, Grants and Contracts for Establishing an Initial Operation; and Section 1204, Grants and Contracts for Expansion and Improvement.

To date, the EMSS Act of 1973 and its amendments have funded programs as shown on the chart, see p. 3.

So far, more than $180 million have been granted for EMSS. It is understandable that federal support cannot last forever. The philosophy, nowadays, is that the federal dollars are only "seed" money. EMSSs have to look for ways to become "self-reliant" in order to survive in the future without federal "transfusions."

Overview

EMS Act Funded Programs

Section of Act	Regions	$ Amount	Population Served
		Fiscal Year 1974	
1202	90	2,250,000	63,000,000
1203	27	10,400,000	18,900,000
1204	9	4,350,000	6,300,000
Total	126	17,000,000	82,200,000
		Fiscal Year 1975	
1202	82	4,617,800	57,400,000
1203	66	19,500,000	46,200,000
1204	26	8,125,000	18,200,000
Total	174	32,242,800	121,800,000
		Fiscal Year 1976	
1203	51	21,836,475	35,700,000
1204	12	7,278,825	8,400,000
Total	63	29,115,300	44,100,000
		Fiscal Year 1977	
1202	23	986,583	16,100,000
1203	54	21,587,304	37,800,000
1204	21	9,716,133	14,700,000
Total	98	32,290,000	68,600,000
		Fiscal Year 1978	
1202	14	870,000	9,800,000
1203	61	23,435,991	42,700,000
1204	25	11,408,009	17,500,000
Total	100	35,714,000	70,000,000
		Fiscal Year 1979	
1202	23	1,129,783	7,700,000
1203	49	20,484,168	34,300,000
1204	33	13,886,049	23,100,000
Total	105	35,500,000	65,100,000[2]

---

2. David R. Boyd, "Emergency Medical Services Systems Development: A National Initiative," IEEE Transactions on Vehicular Technology VT-25 (November 1976): 104-15.

Overview

C. LEGISLATION

We have seen that federal legislation provided the initial impetus for EMS. These basic acts are:

1. The National Highway Safety Act, 1966 (DOT)

2. The Emergency Medical Services Systems Act, 1973 (PL 93-154).
    Amended October 21, 1976 (PL 94-573). Amended December 12, 1979 (PL 96-142)

The EMSS Act (1973, 1976, 1979) is better understood by consulting:

3. "Grants for Emergency Medical Services Systems: Rules and Regulations." Federal Register 43 (3 November 1978): 51532-544.

4. The Emergency Medical Services Systems Program Guidelines. DHEW (HSA) Publication no. 79-2002. West Hyattsville, Md.: U.S. Department of Health, Education and Welfare, Division of Emergency Medical Services, August 1979. 138 p.

At the state level, legislation issues are more complicated. Although 60 percent of the states have some kind of legislation relating to some aspects of EMS, there is no unity or sense of unity of purpose and/or standardization. It is important to point out that the more similarities that exist between states' legislation, the better the cooperation enabled among across-state-line systems in the basic aspect of mutual aid, especially with reference to licensure and certification, and communication linkages.

State laws cover the whole spectrum of EMSS aspects, with emphasis on: emergency medical technician-ambulance training and certification; EMT-paramedic training and certification; levy of taxes to support ambulance services and/or EMS; communicatons; fees for ambulance services; and the Good Samaritan Law.

In order to obtain the latest information on a state's legislation, the best procedure is to contact the State Office of Emergency Medical Services (see appendix).

Chapter 2
SOURCES

A. INFORMATION CENTERS

5. Emergency Care Information Center
    701 Ridgefield Road
    Wilton, Conn. 06897
    (203) 762-3911

    Begun in 1973, Emergency Care Information Center is a private organization devoted to the collection and dissemination of information to serve the needs of EMS professionals and paraprofessionals. The center was organized to satisfy the need for a central source of EMS information, and to communicate this information to the user through responsive and timely publications. Its main publications are: Medical 911 and EMS Communicator. The purpose of Medical 911 is to provide a single current reference to the spectrum of information, materials, and organized support that is available to assist the EMS provider.

6. Emergency Medical Services Information Center (EMSIC)
    American College of Emergency Physicians
    3900 Capital City Boulevard
    Lansing, Mich. 48906
    (517) 321-7911

    This information center was established in 1974 to identify bibliographic materials related to EMS and to provide current accessible resources and reference services to EMS providers, planners, and researchers. EMSIC participates in a computer-based information system developed to produce rapid bibliographic access to EMS literature. EMSIC resources include: (1) medical indexes to EMS literature; (2) a serials collection that includes over one hundred journal titles and sixty EMS related newsletters; (3) a document collection consisting of clinical, EMS systems, socioeconomic and general reference texts; and (4) a vertical file collection with selected bibliographies prepared by EMSIC, publications, audiovisual catalogs, sample ED records, and forms. EMSIC services are: (1) ready reference; (2) selected bibliographies; (3) comprehensive literature search; (4) MEDLINE access; and (5) reproduction of research materials.

Sources

7. National Clearinghouse for Emergency Medical Services
   Division of Emergency Medical Services
   Prince George's Center
   6525 Belcrest Road
   West Hyattsville, Md. 20782
   (301) 436-6267

   > The clearinghouse was established after the interest created by the passage of the Emergency Medical Services Systems Act of 1973 to gather and disseminate the most current information available on EMS. Capabilities include: on-line automated bibliographic information resource; collection of more than ten thousand catalogued and indexed items on EMS subjects, including congressional hearings, reports, research studies, surveys, journal articles, and related documents; and response to mail and telephone inquiries on the full range of emergency medical services subjects.

8. National Emergency Medical Services Information Clearinghouse (NEMSIC)
   Center for the Study of Emergency Health Services
   University of Pennsylvania
   3609 Locust Walk
   Philadelphia, Pa. 19104
   (215) 243-6304

   > NEMSIC was established in 1973 with funds provided by the ACT Foundation and funds provided by the Robert Wood Johnson Foundation. It is operated by the Center for the Study of Emergency Health Services, University of Pennsylvania. Its main purpose is to gather and deliver information to persons and organizations working in the field of emergency medical services systems.

B. BIBLIOGRAPHIES

9. Afifi, M., et al., comps. <u>Bibliography of Emergency Medical Services Literature Obtained from Computer Indexed Information Sources.</u> Los Angeles: University of Southern California, Western Research Application Center, July 1974. 70 p. (Available from NTIS, Springfield, Va. 22161. PB-238 852.

   > The search of "Emergency medical service" was conducted against MEDLINE GRA, NASA, and ERIC data banks covering the period from 1969 to the present. This search has produced much relevant information which can be found in this report under the following categories: system design; data collection; information management; trauma; education and training; standards, criteria, guidelines, and evaluation; facilities; communication; and transportation.

10. Cohen, Susan. <u>Emergency Care Bibliography.</u> New York: Columbia University, Faculty of Medicine, Center for Community Health Systems, May 1972. 66 p.

Sources

This annotated bibliography of articles and publications relating to emergency services was compiled to identify the work of others that could provide relevant facts and insights for studying emergency services. It is a working document. The references are cross-indexed by author and subject area. There are ten subject area groupings. The first nine correspond to the critical problem areas associated with emergency services identified by the center's emergency services project team. They include: patterns of seeking care; patient flow and management; space; information systems; staffing of emergency services; economics of emergency services; administrative structures and managerial procedures; comprehensive care in emergency services; and services outside of hospital. The tenth grouping is composed of references which provide overviews of the emergency services system. There is also a listing of not readily available material relevant to the subject area which has not been abstracted. (Author's introduction)

11. Hamilton, William F., and William, Thomas J., comps. <u>Emergency Health System Planning: An Annotated Bibliography.</u> Philadelphia: Center for the Study of Emergency Health Services and the Leonard Davis Institute of Health Economics, 1973. 70 p.

   The purpose of this bibliography is to provide planners and others interested in emergency medical services with a useful summary of previously reported efforts in organizing and operating EMS systems. Selected references in this field have been organized according to the following general phases of system planning and development: (1) organizational activities: setting up EMS councils and seeking funds; (2) descriptive studies: describing the current EMS system so that areas of potential improvement can be identified; (3) system design: (a) specifying EMS goals, (b) identifying alternatives for system improvement, (c) methodologies for evaluating prospective changes to determine which alternative offers the most improvement, (d) applications of evaluation methodologies; and (4) implementation.

12. Harrison, Elizabeth A., comp. <u>Biotelemetry: A Bibliography With Abstracts.</u> Springfield, Va.: NTIS, January 1975. 139 p. (PS-75/094)

   The bibliography contains 139 selected abstracts. It includes reports which cover biomedical information systems, biometeorology, animal and bird migrations, bioinstrumentation, electrocardiography, ecology, and electroencephalography as related to biotelemetry.

13. _____. <u>Emergency Medical Services: Costs. A Bibliography with Abstracts.</u> Springfield, Va.: NTIS, October 1977. 43 p. (PS-77/0904)

   Cost effectiveness of medical equipment, recommendations for reducing costs, and methodology for estimating financial impact of emergency medical services systems is covered by the selected citations. Analysis, estimations, and projections of costs

Sources

are discussed as related to models, resources, legislation, government funds, outcomes measurement, financing, and operations.

14. _____. Emergency Medical Services: Health Planning. A Bibliography With Abstracts. Springfield, Va.: NTIS, October 1977. 65 p. (PS-77/0905)

    Communication, training, transportation, emergency care facilities, and community education for rural and urban areas are included. The reports discuss plan implementation and plan development for states and regions. Ambulance and hospital emergency services are also discussed.

15. _____. Emergency Medical Services: Hospitals. A Bibliography With Abstracts. Springfield, Va.: NTIS, October 1977. 37 p. (PS-77/0907)

    Categorization, workload, resources, capabilities, assessments, financial impact, planning, and implementation of hospital emergency medical services are the subjects covered. Citations discussing policy and procedure guidelines, surveys, and training of personnel are included.

16. _____. Emergency Medical Services: Rural Areas. A Bibliography With Abstracts. Springfield, Va.: NTIS, October 1977. 40 p. (PS-77/0903)

    Transportation, planning, management, medical equipment, and education as related to emergency medical services in rural areas are included in the selection. The bibliography also covers health manpower, health resources, costs, and health care delivery.

17. _____. Emergency Medical Services: Transportation. A Bibliography With Abstracts. Springfield, Va.: NTIS, October 1977. 50 p. (PS-77/0906)

    Air and ground transportation for rural and urban areas is covered. Some abstracts discuss the evaluation and planning of emergency medical service systems, using systems analysis and mathematical models. Specific subjects covered are helicopter ambulances, coronary care units, and military assistance to safety and traffic. Capital requirements and operating costs are also included.

18. _____. Emergency Medical Services: Utilization. A Bibliography With Abstracts. Springfield, Va.: NTIS, October 1977. 61 p. (PS-77/0902)

    Predicting demand, utilization patterns, extent of utilization, and resources utilized are subjects covered. The specific facilities discussed are hospital emergency departments, health maintenance organizations, neighborhood health centers, and ambulance services. Attitudes and surveys related to utilization of emergency medical services are included.

Sources

19. _____. Emergency Medical Services and Care: A Bibliography with Abstracts. Springfield, Va.: NTIS, January 1975. 87 p. (PS-75/71)

    The selected citations include outpatient services, intensive care units, hospital administration, hospital emergency rooms, medical personnel, telecommunication, traffic safety, and training as related to emergency medical services and care.

20. _____. Health Care Delivery: A Bibliography with Abstracts. Springfield, Va.: NTIS, May 1975. 137 p.

    Government-sponsored reports cover research and evaluation of health care delivery systems for rural and urban populations. Information is reported on regional and community medical programs, the economics of health care delivery systems, health maintenance organizations, emergency medical care, biomedical information systems, and ambulatory health care.

21. _____. Health Services in Rural Areas: A Bibliography with Abstracts. Springfield, Va.: NTIS, June 1975. 87 p. (PS-75/532)

    The selected abstracts of federally sponsored research reports cover telecommunication, rehabilitation, emergency medical programs, medical education, health care delivery, medical personnel, and medical facilities in rural areas.

22. _____. Telecommunications in Medicine: A Bibliography with Abstracts. Springfield, Va.: NTIS, July 1975. 41 p. (PS-75/580)

    These selected citations of federally sponsored research reports cover teleconsultation, communications for emergency medical services, medical communication networks, and television systems, and rural health services.

23. National Library of Medicine. The Hospital Emergency Room: 194 Citations in English. Rockville, Md.: January 1970 through June 1973. 11 p. (Literature Search No. 73-26)

    The emphasis of the bibliography is on the education of emergency room physician and nurse, medicolegal implications, and also the planning, standardization, quality, and utilization of the service. Arranged in alphabetical order by authors. No index.

24. Noble, John H., Jr., et al., eds. Emergency Medical Services: Selected Bibliography. New York: Behavioral Publications, 1974. 147 p.

    There are over twelve-hundred items in this bibliography whose sources are: (1) articles cited in the main volume (EMS, 1973); (2) MEDLINE searches; and (3) review of the existing literature. It is divided into five main parts: (1) the emergency medical system; (2) patterns of emergency room utilization; (3) transportation and communications;

Sources

(4) standards and policies; and (5) other bibliographies and collections. No index.

25. Padget, Virginia, ed. <u>Emergency Medical Services Bibliography.</u> Washington, D.C.: National Highway Traffic Safety Administration, Office of Administrative Services, Technical Reference Division, 1974. 100 p.

> This bibliography contains 453 annotated entries. Citations have been previously published in the <u>Highway Safety Literature.</u> This source contains good information, but it is hard to use because it lacks an index.

26. Plaas, Hyrum, et al., eds. <u>The Evaluation of Policy Related Research in Emergency Medical Services: A Selected and Critical Annotated Bibliography.</u> 4 vols. Knoxville: University of Tennessee, Bureau of Public Administration, August 30, 1974.

> This bibliography has been prepared to provide an assessment and critical review of a large number of studies and research which have been undertaken in EMS. It reflects the field of research which we have been able to identify, collect, read, and critically review since September 1973. Research included in the bibliography fulfills the following broad requirements: (1) It was a research undertaking in that information was systematically assembled and it was data-based. (2) It focused on some aspect of emergency medical services, its components and environments. (3) It provided methodology which may be used by others to provide information concerning policy alternatives and the conditions under which decisions can be made. (Author's introduction)

27. Reed, William E., comp. <u>Land Mobile Communication: A Bibliography with Abstracts.</u> Springfield, Va.: NTIS, July 1975. 51 p. (PS-75/546)

> The cited federally sponsored research reports include topics on public policy, frequency allocation and management, licensee data, satellite relays, propagation, and forecasts.

28. _____. <u>Portable Radio Equipment: A Bibliography with Abstracts.</u> Springfield, Va.: NTIS, July 1975. 65 p. (PS-75/547)

> Federally sponsored research is cited on portable transmitters, receivers, antennas, power sources, and components. Reports on wave propagation of portable radio equipment are included.

29. U.S. Department of Health, Education and Welfare. Division of Emergency Health Services. <u>Emergency Health Services Selected Bibliography.</u> Emergency Health Series, A-1. Rockville, Md.: 1970. 175.

> The bibliography is divided into four main sections. Part 1 has publications that deal with day-to-day health emergencies that occur at home, at work, and at play. Examples are strokes, heart attacks, and injuries from roadside accidents.

Sources

Part 2 lists documents that will help communities to prepare for major emergencies, including national disasters and nuclear war. Part 3 lists films and slides on disaster care and includes a special instructional kit to train people in medical self-help when a doctor cannot be reached. Part 4 provides sources of catalogs, bibliographies, and publications lists that include material on disaster care and day-to-day health emergencies.

30. U.S. Department of Health, Education and Welfare. Division of Emergency Medical Services. Categorization of Hospital Emergency Services: Selected Bibliography. DHEW Publication no. (HSA) 76-2026. West Hyattsville, Md.: 1976. 15 p.

    The twenty-five items in this bibliography, with abstracts, are the best known works in the area of categorization. This material should enable planners to gain insight into the potential advantages which categorization can bring to EMS.

31. _____. Rural Emergency Medical Services: Selected Bibliography. DHEW Publication no. (HSA) 76-2028. West Hyattsville, Md.: 1976. 24 p.

    This bibliography shows the different viewpoints in implementing a rural EMS system. The strongest pattern recommended is that in which there is a cooperation of local resources through an EMS council that shall coordinate all available resources.

32. U.S. Department of Transporation. National Highway Traffic Safety Administration. Office of Administrative Services. Technical Reports of the National Highway Traffic Safety Administration: A Bibliography 1967-1972. Washington, D.C.: n.d. 360 p. (DOT HS-820 252)

    The technical reports of the NHTSA which are cited in this bibliography are the product of research and testing that fulfill objectives of the administration in the fields of highway and motor vehicle safety.

33. U.S. Department of Transportation. National Highway Traffic Safety Administration. Office of Management Systems. Emergency Medical Services: A Bibliography with Abstracts. Special Bibliography, no. 8. Washington, D.C.: May 1974. 103 p.

    The documents cited are in the NHTSA Technical Services Division collection and can be examined there. Since this collection was established in 1967, most of the publications bear a publication date of 1967 or later. Citations and abstracts are those that have previously appeared in the NHTSA publication, Highway Safety Literature.

34. Use of Helicopters for Air Delivery and Emergency: A DDC Bibliography. Alexandria, Va.: Defense Documentation Center, Cameron Station, March 1975. 39 p. (NTIS AD-A 006 750)

Sources

This bibliography contains citations of thirty-nine unclassified reports dealing with use of helicopters for air delivery and emergency, aerial delivery, air drop operations, search and rescue, and emergency medical care.

C. COMPUTERIZED DATA BASE

The application of computer technology to information management has facilitated the task of the person searching for adequate data. The easiest and quickest way to initiate a bibliographic search, especially for the neophyte, is to locate a good library, preferably a regional medical library or university library with computer retrieval capability. Some computerized data sources are:

>Emergency Medical Services Information Center (EMSIC)
>American College of Emergency Physicians
>3900 Capital City Boulevard
>Lansing, Mich. 48906
>(517) 321-7911

>Institute for Scientific Information
>3501 Market Street
>Philadelphia, Pa. 19104
>(215) 386-0100

>National Clearinghoue for Emergency Medical Services
>Division of Emergency Medical Services
>6525 Belcrest Road
>West Hyattsville, Md. 29782
>(301) 436-6267

>National Library of Medicine or Regional Medical Library
>8600 Rockville Pike
>Bethesda, Md. 20014

>National Technical Information Service
>5285 Port Royal Road
>Springfield, Va. 22151

D. PERIODICALS

The researcher can follow the theoretical and practical developments in the field of EMS in periodical publications (journals and newsletters).

There are journals published by professional associations, such as the American Association of Emergency Physicians (<u>Annals of Emergency Medicine</u>), American Association for the Surgery of Trauma (<u>Journal of Trauma</u>). Commercial enterprises issue <u>Emergency Medical Services, Emergency, Fire Engineering,</u> and <u>Medical 911.</u> Newsletters originate from diverse sources. <u>EMS Communicator</u> is a product of a private venture, as is the <u>EMT Legal Bulletin.</u> Many associations publish their bulletins or newsletters, such as, <u>International Rescuer,</u> and <u>Traumagram.</u> Most state EMS offices have their own newsletters.

To keep the historical perspective, we are also including titles that have ceased publication.

Sources

Journals

35. AAAM QUARTERLY JOURNAL. 1969-- . Ed. Norman E. McSwain. American Association for Automotive Medicine, P.O. Box 222, Morton Grove, III. 60053.

36. ACCIDENT FACTS. Annual. Managing Ed. J.L. Recht. National Safety Council, 444 North Michigan Avenue, Chicago, III. 60611.

37. AID. 1974-- . Monthly. Ambulance Association of America, 1629 K Street, N.W., Washington, D.C. 20006.

38. AMBULANCE JOURNAL. 1973-- . Monthly. Ambulance Service Institute, Association of Chief Ambulance Officers, National Institute of Ambulance Instructors, 79 Dudbury Avenue, Ferndown, Dorset BH22 8DY, Great Britain.

39. ANNALS OF EMERGENCY MEDICINE. 1979-- . Monthly. Ed. N.E. Perkin. Formerly: Journal of the American College of Emergency Physicians. 1972-79. American College of Emergency Physicians, 3900 Capital City Boulevard, Lansing, Mich. 48906. (517) 321-7911.

40. BULLETIN OF THE AMERICAN COLLEGE OF SURGEONS. 1915-- . Monthly. Ed. Dennis M. Connauphton. American College of Surgeons, 55 East Erie Street, Chicago, III. 60611. (312) 664-4050.

41. CANADIAN EMERGENCY SERVICES NEWS. 1978-- . Bimonthly. Ed. Harold Gunderson. 2116 Twenty-Seventh Avenue, N.E., Calgary, Alberta T2E 7A6, Canada.

42. CRITICAL CARE MEDICINE. 1973-- . Bimonthly. Ed. William C. Shoennken. Official Journal of the Society of Critical Care Medicine, William and Wilkins, 428 East Preston Street, Baltimore, Md. 21202.

43. CRITICAL CARE UPDATE. 1974-- . Monthly. Ed. Donna Zschoche. National Critical Care Institute of Education, P.O. Box 5827, Orange, Calif. 92667.

44. EMERGENCY. 1969-- . Bimonthly. Ed. Rick Minerd. Dyna Graphics, P.O. Box 159, Carlsbad, Calif. 92008. (714) 438-2511.

45. EMERGENCY DEPARTMENT NEWS, 5622 Columbia Pike, Suite 204, Falls Church, Va. 22041. (703) 998-5411.

46. EMERGENCY HEALTH SERVICES QUARTERLY. 1980-- . Ed. Michael Pozen. Boston Coty Hospital, 818 Harrison Avenue, Boston, Mass. 02118.

Sources

47. EMERGENCY MEDICAL SERVICES. 1969-- . Bimonthly. Ed. Joan Hart. 12849 Magnolia Boulevard, North Hollywood, Calif. 91607. (213) 980-4184.

48. EMERGENCY MEDICAL SERVICES DIGEST, Washington Fire News Service, 7620 Little River Turnpike, Annandale, Va. 22003. (703) 941-6600.

49. EMERGENCY MEDICINE. 1969-- . Monthly. Ed. Irving J. Cohen. 280 Madison Avenue, New York, N.Y. 10016. (212) 889-4530.

50. EMERGENCY NURSE LEGAL BULLETIN. 1975-- . Quarterly. Ed. James E. George. MED/LAW Publishers, P.O. Box 293, Westville, N.J. 08093.

51. EMERGENCY PHYSICIAN LEGAL BULLETIN. 1978-- . Quarterly. Ed. James E. George. MED/LAW Publishers, P.O. Box 293, Westville, N.J. 08093.

52. EMERGENCY PRODUCT NEWS, GHP Publications, P.O. Box 926, Encinitas, Calif. 92024. (714) 753-6475.

53. EMT JOURNAL. 1977-- . Quarterly. Ed. J.D. Farrington. C.V. Mosby Co., Circulation Department, 11830 Westline Industrial Drive, St. Louis, Mo. 63141.

54. FIRE COMMAND. 1933-- . Monthly. Ed. Joyce Keefe. National Fire Protection Association, 60 Batterymarch, Boston, Mass. 02110.

55. FIRE ENGINEERING. 1877-- . Monthly. Ed. James F. Corey. 666 Fifth Avenue, New York, N.Y. 10019.

56. HEART AND LUNG, THE JOURNAL OF CRITICAL CARE. Bimonthly. Ed. Dorothy M. Voorman. Official Publication of American Association of Critical Care Nurses, C.V. Mosby Co., Circulation Department, 11830 Westline Industrial Drive, St. Louis, Mo. 63141.

57. INJURY. 1969-- . Bimonthly. Ed. R.L. Batten. John Wright and Sons, 42-44 Triangle W., Bristol, England; and Williams and Wilkins, 428 East Preston Street, Baltimore, Md. 21201.

58. INTERNATIONAL RESCUER. 1947-- . Bimonthly. Ed. L.L. Weber. International Rescuer and First Aid Association, 5201 Madison Road, Cincinnati, Ohio 45227.

59. INTERRESCUE INFORMATION, A.I.S.S., Statenlaan 81, The Hague, Netherlands.

Sources

60. JOURNAL OF EMERGENCY MEDICAL SERVICES (JEMS). 1976-- . Monthly. Ed. James O. Page. Formerly: Paramedics International, P.O. Box 152, Morristown, N.J. 07960. (201) 766-7937.

61. JOURNAL OF EMERGENCY NURSING (JEN). 1978-- . Bimonthly. Ed. Janet Barber. 666 North Lake Shore Drive, Chicago, Ill. 60611. (312) 649-0297.

62. JOURNAL OF TRAFFIC MEDICINE. 1973-- . Quarterly. Ed. Rune Andreasson. International Association for Accident and Traffic Medicine, 535 North Dearborn Street, Chicago, Ill 60610. (312) 751-6000; and Box 10043, 5-100, Stockholm, 10, Sweden.

63. JOURNAL OF TRAUMA. 1961-- . Monthly. Ed. John H. Davis. Williams and Wilkins, 428 East Preston Street, Baltimore, Md. 21202.

64. JOURNAL OF WINTER EMERGENCY CARE. 1975-- . 3 per year. Ed. Betty Kleiner. National Ski Patrol System, 5 Flintlock Ridge, Simsbury, Conn. 06070. (203) 658-5670.

65. MEDICAL 911. 1973-- . Bimonthly. Ed. Thomas Wetzel. Emergency Care Information Center, 701 Ridgefield Road, Wilton, Conn. 06897. (203) 762-3911.

66. MINNESOTA FIRE CHIEF. 1964-- . Bimonthly. Minnesota State Fire Chiefs' Association, 4141 Harriet Avenue, Minneapolis, Minn. 55409.

67. NATIONAL SAFETY NEWS. 1919-- . Monthly. Ed. Roy Fisher. National Safety Council, 444 North Fischer Avenue, Chicago, Ill. 60611. (312) 527-4800.

68. OCCUPATIONAL HEALTH AND SAFETY. Bimonthly. Ed. Carl Zenz. P.O. Box 7573, Waco, Tex. 76710. (817) 752-6566.

69. PARA-MEDICAL JOURNAL. 1968-- . Quarterly. Pennsylvania Ambulance Association, Weamer Building, Room 23, 15 South Seventh Street, Indiana, Pa. 15701.

70. RESPONSE, Quarterly. Ed. Wayne Jenkins. Institute of Ambulance Officers, P.O. Box 46, Lancefield, Australia 3435.

71. REVIEW. Ambulance and Medical Services Association of America, P.O. Box 14178, Hartford, Conn. 06114.

72. SCI DIGEST. Quarterly. Ed. Delman McNeil. National Spinal Cord Injury Data Research Center, 1130 East McDowell Road, Suite A-6, Phoenix, Ariz. 85006. (602) 257-4222.

Sources

73. SEARCH AND RESCUE MAGAZINE. 4195 Polaris Avenue, Lompoe, Calif. 93436. (805) 733-3986.

74. SPOKESMAN, Ambulance Society of America, 230 East Fifth Street, St. Paul, Minn. 55101.

75. STAT. Quarterly. Ed. Robert T. Fitzgerald. 1520 Arizona, Santa Monica, Calif. 90404. (213) 451-0783.

76. TOPICS IN EMERGENCY MEDICINE. 1979-- . Quarterly. Aspen Systems Corp., 20010 Century Boulevard, Germantown, Md. 20767. (301) 428-0700.

77. TRAFFIC SAFETY. 1927-- . Monthly. Ed. Angela Maher. National Safety Council, 444 North Michigan Avenue, Chicago, Ill. 60611. (312) 527-4800.

Newsletters

78. AAOS EMS NEWSLETTER. Quarterly. Ed. Swan Nowicki. American Academy of Orthopaedic Surgeons, 444 North Michigan Avenue, Chicago, Ill. 60611. (312) 822-0970.

79. AMSAA NEWSLETTER. 1975-- . Irregular. Ambulance and Medical Services Association of America, P.O. Box 14178, Hartford, Conn. 06114. (203) 522-8690.

80. AMSAA PARAMEDICAL NEWS REVIEW. Ambulance and Medical Services Association of America, P.O. Box 14178, Hartford, Conn. 06114. (203) 522-8690.

81. ACCIDENT REPORTER. 1974-- . Monthly. University of North Carolina, Highway Safety Research Center, Chapel Hill, N.C. 27514.

82. ALABAMA RESCUER. 1965-- . Quarterly. Ed. G.B. Casey. 1115 Walnut Street, Gadsden, Ala. 39501. (205) 547-3175.

83. BAY AREA EMS PRESS. Association of Bay Area Governments, Hotel Claremont, Berkeley, Calif. 94705. (415) 841-9730.

84. BLANKET. Quarterly. Ed. John Robortella. New York State Volunteer Ambulance and First Aid Association, 47 Lansing Circle, Rochester, N.Y. 14624. (716) 436-1200.

85. BURN FOUNDATION NEWSLETTER. 1974-- . Monthly. 250 South Seventeenth Street, Philadelphia, Pa. 19103.

86. CARDIAC ALERT. Monthly. Ed. Toni Weiss. 8 Bluestone Terrace, Morristown, N.J. 07960. (201) 538-7938.

Sources

87. CENTRAL MASSACHUSETTS EMS NEWS. Ed. Don LeBlanc. 55 Lake Avenue, North Worcester, Mass. 01605. (617) 798-0755.

88. CIVIL AIR PATROL NEWS. Ed. Frank Lowry. Maxwell AFB, Ala. 36112.

89. COLORADO SEARCH AND RESCUE BOARD BULLETIN. 2415 East Maplewood Avenue, Littleton, Colo. 80121. (203) 794-2304.

90. COMMUNITY EMERGENCY CARE NEWSLETTER. c/o US PHS Hospital, 14 Fifteenth Avenue and Luke Street, San Francisco, Calif. 94118. (415) 752-1400, Ext. 323.

91. DELAWARE PROVIDER. Delaware Office of EMS, Dover, Del. 19901. (302) 678-4710.

92. DIVE RESCUE JOURNAL. International Association of Dive Rescue Specialists, 1449 Riverside Drive, Fort Collins, Colo. 80524.

93. EDNA ROADRUNNER. Emergency Department Nurses Association, 666 North Lake Shore Drive, Chicago, Ill. 60611. (312) 649-0297.

94. EMERGENCY CARE NEWS. 1974-- . Monthly. Ed. Jim Malone. EMS/Technical Assistance Program, Public Technology, 1140 Connecticut Avenue, N.W., Washington, D.C. 20036. (202) 223-8240.

95. EMERGENCY HEALTH SERVICES BULLETIN. Pennsylvania Department of Health, Division of Emergency Health Services, P.O. Box 90, Harrisburg, Pa. 17120.

96. EMERGENCY HEALTH SERVICES IN NEW YORK STATE. New York State Department of Health, Health Facilities and Preventive Services Program, 2 Bureau of Emergency Health Services, 84 Holland Avenue, Albany, N.Y. 12208.

97. EMERGENCY MEDICAL SERVICES BRIEF. EMS Production Manager, Control Data Corporation, Application and Professional Division, 901 South Highland Street, Arlington, Va. 22204.

98. EMERGENCY MEDICAL SERVICES DISPATCH. Bimonthly. Emergency Health Services Federation of South Central Pennsylvania, 3524 Trindle Road, Camp Hill, Pa. 17011. (717) 763-0730.

99. EMERGENCY MEDICAL SERVICES NEWS OF THE MONTH. State of Florida, Department of Health and Rehabilitative Services, Division of Health, Emergency Medical Services Section, P.O. Box 210, Jacksonville, Fla. 32201.

100 EMERGENCY MEDICINE RESIDENCY NEWSLETTER. 1972-- . 3900 Capitol City Boulevard, Lansing, Mich. 48906.

Sources

101. EMERGENCY MEDICINE TODAY. 1972-75. Monthly. American Medical Association, Commission on EMS, 535 North Dearborn Street, Chicago III. 60610.

102. EMS ACCESS. Quarterly. Ed. Jim Parker. EMS Section, Minnesota Department of Health, 717 Delaware Street, S.E., Minneapolis, Minn. 55440. (612) 296-5281.

103. EMS ACTION. 1977-- . Monthly. ACT Foundation, Basking Ridge, N.J. 07920.

104. EMS COMMUNICATOR. Indiana EMS Commission, 315 State Office Building, Indianapolis, Ind. 46204. (317) 633-4055.

105. EMS COMMUNICATOR. Bimonthly. Ed. Thomas Wetzel. Emergency Care Information Center, 701 Ridgefield Road, Wilton, Conn. 06897. (203) 762-3911.

106. EMS DISPATCH. 1975-- . Irregular. North Central Connecticut EMS, 97 Elm Street, Hartford, Conn. 06106. (203) 249-7601.

107. EMSI NEWSLETTER. 1976-- . Monthly. Ed. Susan Lambert. Emergency Medical Services Institute, 564 Forbes Avenue, Pittsburgh, Pa. 15219. (412) 562-1843.

108. EMS INFORMER. Quarterly. Ed. Wade Spruill. EMS Division, Mississippi State Board of Health, P.O. Box 1700, Jackson, Miss. 39205. (601) 982-6608.

109. EMS NEWS. Monthly. Ed. Bennie Lou Carr. Georgia Emergency Health Section, 618 Ponce de Leon Avenue, Atlanta, Ga. 30380. (404) 894-5170.

110. EMS NEWS. Bimonthly. Ed. Vijay R. Sudersanam. North Carolina Office of EMS, P.O. Box 12200, Raleigh, N.C. 27605. (919) 733-2285.

111. EMS NEWS. (Westchester County, N.Y.) 1975-- . Irregular. 148 Martine Avenue, Room 228A, White Plains, N.Y. 10601. (914) 682-2707.

112. EMS NEWSLETTER. 1973-- . Monthly. Arizona Department of Public Safety, Division of EMS, P.O. Box 6638, Phoenix, Ariz. 85005.

113. EMS NEWSLETTER. 1973-- . Monthly. Connecticut Advisory Committee on EMS, 79 Elm Street, Room 227, Hartford, Conn. 06115.

114. EMS NEWSLETTER. Quarterly. South Cook County EMSS, One Ingalls Drive, Harvey, III. 60426. (312) 333-2300.

Sources

115. EMS NEWSLETTER. 1974-- . Irregular. Maryland Department of Health and Mental Hygiene, Division of Emergency Medical Services, 22 South Greene Street, Baltimore, Md. 21201.

116. EMS NEWSLETTER. Monthly. Ed. John Hubinger. Michigan Department of Public Health, EMS Section, 3500 North Logan, Lansing, Mich. 48909. (517) 373-1406.

117. EMS NEWSLETTER. 1974-- . Bimonthly. Emergency Medical Services Bureau, 1424 Ninth Avenue, Helena, Mont. 59601.

118. EMS NEWSLETTER. Regional Emergency Medical Service of Northwest Ohio, P.O. Box 6190, Medical College of Ohio, Toledo, Ohio 43614.

119. EMS NEWSLETTER. Bimonthly. Bureau of EMS, 109 Governor Street, Richmond, Va. 23219. (904) 786-5188.

120. EMS NEW YORK. Bimonthly. Ed. Linda Heinzelman. EMS Systems Development, Twenty-First Street and First Avenue, New York, N.Y. 10010. (212) 685-0088.

121. EMS NORTHWEST. EMS Council of Northwestern Pennsylvania, 1545 West Thirty-Eighth Street, Erie, Pa. 16508. (814) 864-0634.

122. EMS OKLAHOMA. Oklahoma Highway Safety Office, Oklahoma City, Okla. 73105. (405) 521-3314.

123. EMS REGION REPORT. North Alabama EMS, P.O. Box 2104, Decatur, Ala. 35602.

124. EMS RESOURCE BULLETIN. Quarterly. Ed. Michael P. Olsen. U.S. Fire Administration, Washington, D.C. 20472. (202) 634-7663.

125. EMS RESPONSE TIME. Northern California Emergency Medical Care Council, 630 Azalea Avenue, Redding, Calif. 96001.

126. EMSS REPORTS. 1976-- . Bimonthly. Emergency Medical Services Section, Oregon State Health Division, Room 905, Cascade Building, 520 Southwest Sixth Avenue, Portland, Oreg. 97204.

127. EMS TRANSMITTER. Los Angeles County Office of EMS, 313 North Figueroa, Los Angeles, Calif. 90012. (213) 874-8144.

128. EMT LEGAL BULLETIN. Quarterly. Ed. James E. George. MED/LAW Publishers, P.O. Box 293, Westville, N.J. 08093.

129. EMT NEWS. Bimonthly. Ed. Larry Menkes. EMTS of Connecticut, P.O. Box 57, Stratford, Conn. 06497. (203) 227-1134.

Sources

130. EMT NEWSLETTER. C.V. Mosby Co., 11830 Westline Industrial Drive, St. Louis, Mo. 63141.

131. FIRST AID BULLETIN. 1947-- . Monthly. Virginia Association of Volunteer Rescue Squads. Ed. J.E. Adams. 1406 Norcross, Lynchburg, Va. 24502.

132. FORESIGHT. Defense Civil Preparedness Agency, The Pentagon, Washington, D.C. 20301.

133. GOLD CROSS. New Jersey First Aid Council. Harry Van Buskirk. Circulation Manager, 11 Semel Avenue, Iselin, N.J. 08830. (201) 549-8417.

134. HIGHWAY LOSS REDUCTION STATUS REPORT. Biweekly. Ed. Paul C. Hood. Insurance Institute for Highway Safety, Washington, D.C. 20037. (202) 333-0770.

135. IAATM NEWSLETTER. International Association for Accidental and Traffic Medicine. 535 North Dearborn Street, Chicago, Ill. 60610. (312) 751-6000.

136. ILLINOIS EMS NEWS. Illinois Department of Public Health. Division of EMS and Highway Safety, 535 West Jefferson Street, Springfield, Ill. 62761.

137. INFORMATION DIGEST. Division of EMS, Nebraska Department of Health, P.O. Box 95007, Lincoln, Nebr. 68509. (402) 471-2158.

138. INTERNATIONAL RESCUER. Quarterly. Ed. Lodge Weber. International Rescue and Emergency Care Association, 3200 Valleyview Drive, Columbus, Ohio 43204. (614) 274-7750.

139. IPR NEWSLETTER. MIT. Operation Research Center, Room 4-209, Innovative Resource Planning in Urban and Public Safety Systems, Cambridge, Mass. 02139. (617) 253-1356.

140. KEMTA NEWS. Bimonthly. Ed. Vickie Dyck. Kansas Emergency Medical Technicians Association, P.O. Box 744, Newton, Kans. 67114. (316) 283-5894.

141. MAINE EMS NEWS. Bimonthly. EMS Program, Maine Department of Human Services, Augusta, Maine 04333. (207) 289-2411.

142. MARYLAND EMS NEWS. Quarterly. Ed. Beverly Sopp. Maryland Institute for Emergency Medical Services Systems, 22 South Greene Street, Baltimore, Md. 21201. (301) 528-3697.

143. MARYLAND FIRE AND RESCUE INSTITUTE BULLETIN. 1912-- . Monthly. University of Maryland, College Park, Md. 20742.

Sources

144. MARYLAND RESCUE JOURNAL. Quarterly. Ed. Charles Perry. P.O. Box 3052, Baltimore, Md. 21229. (301) 242-5112.

145. MASSACHUSETTS EMS. Monthly. Ed. Bob Buckley. Massachusetts Association of EMTS, P.O. Box 1448, Framingham, Mass. 01701. (617) 358-2721.

146. MASSACHUSETTS EMS ALERT. Massachusetts Department of Public Health, Office of Emergency Medical Services, 600 Washington Street, Room 406, Boston, Mass. 02116. (617) 542-8784.

147. MEDICAL EMERGENCY DISTRICT INTERCOUNTY SERVICES, Garden Court, Alta Vista Road, Louisville, Ky. 40205.

148. MEDIC ALERT NEWSLETTER. 1956-- . Bimonthly. Ed. Dennis Brennen. Medic Alert Foundation, P.O. Box 1009, Turlock, Calif. 95380. (209) 632-2371.

149. MICHIGAN EMERGENCY SERVICES HEALTH COUNCIL NEWS. 1975-- . Bimonthly. 1111 Michigan Avenue, Suite 200, East Lansing, Mich. 48823. (517) 351-0290.

150. MICHIGAN EMT. 8 per year. Ed. John Fick. Michigan Association of EMTs, P.O. Box 1591, Ann Arbor, Mich. 48106. (313) 569-7033.

151. MISSOURI EMERGENCY MEDICAL SERVICES. Bimonthly. Ed. Nancy Hudson. Missouri Bureau of EMS, P.O. Box 570, Jefferson City, Mo. 65102. (314) 751-2713.

152. NAEMT NEWS. Official Publication of the National Association of Emergency Medical Technicians, P.O. Box 334, Newton Highlands, Mass. 02161.

153. NAEP NEWSLETTER. National Association of Emergency Paramedics, 800 West Central Road, Arlington Heights, Ill. 60005. (612) 398-3875.

154. NASAR BRIEFINGS AND GAZETTE. Bimonthly. Ed. Louis Levinson. National Association of Search and Rescue, P.O. Box 2123, LaJolla, Calif. 92038. (714) 268-3266.

155. NATIONAL PATROLLER. Quarterly. Ed. Audrey Adams. National Ski Patrol System, P.O. Box 343, Burlington, Wis. 53105. (414) 763-8844.

156. NEBRASKA EMERGENCY MEDICAL SERVICES ACCESS. Nebraska State Department of Health, Division of Emergency Health Medical Services, 1003 O Street, Lincoln, Nebr. 68508.

157. NEISS NEWS. U.S. Consumer Product Safety Commission, 5401 Westbard Avenue, Bethesda, Md. 20207.

Sources

158. NEWS FROM: REMSNO. Regional EMS of Northwest Ohio, P.O. Box 6190, Toledo, Ohio 43614.

159. NEWS FROM THE HUDSON VALLEY REGIONAL EMERGENCY MEDICAL SERVICES SYSTEM; A MONTHLY BULLETIN. Ed. Monique Hea. c/o Westchester County Health Department, County Office Building, White Plains, N.Y. 10601. (914) 682-2372.

160. NEWSLETTER STATE OF OREGON EMERGENCY MEDICAL SERVICES. Oregon State Health Division, Emergency Medical Services, P.O. Box 231, Portland, Oreg. 97207. (503) 229-5586.

161. NORTH CAROLINA EMERGENCY NEWS. Monthly. Ed. Graham Johnson. 115 Texas Street, Elkin, N.C. 28621. (804) 644-2722.

162. NORTH CAROLINA EMS NEWS. 1974-- . Monthly. North Carolina Department of Human Resources, Office of Emergency Medical Services, P.O. Box 12200, Raleigh, N.C. 27605.

163. NORTH CAROLINA RESCUE NEWS. 1961-- . Monthly. North Carolina Association of Rescue Squads, P.O. Box 553, Greenville, N.C. 27834.

164. NORTH MISSISSIPPI EMS NEWS. Quarterly. Ed. Barbara Criswell. North Mississippi EMS Authority, 116 North Main, Pontotoc, Miss. 38863. (601) 489-2006.

165. NOTICIERO DE EMERGENCIA MEDICA. Commonwealth of Puerto Rico, Department of Health, Secretary of EMS, Santurce, P.R. 00908.

166. OREGON TRAUMA NEWSLETTER. Quarterly. Ed. Joseph Vander Veer, Jr., 6533 Northeast Sandy Boulevard, Portland, Oreg. 97213.

167. PARAMEDIC NEWS. Quarterly. Ed. Ginger Murphy. University Hospital EMS Training Office, 225 Dickinson Street, San Diego, Calif. 92103. (714) 294-6449.

168. PARAMEDIC NEWSLETTER. County of Los Angeles, Department of Health Services, Paramedic Services and Pre-Hospital Care Section, 313 North Figueroa Street, 7th Floor, Los Angeles, Calif. 90012.

169. PENNSYLVANIA AMBULANCE ASSOCIATION NEWSLETTER. Pennsylvania Ambulance Association, Weamer Building, Room 23, 15 South Seventh Street, Indiana, Pa. 15701. (412) 465-2214.

170. PENNSYLVANIA EMERGENCY HEALTH SERVICES COUNCIL NEWSLETTER. Quarterly. Ed. Joel Grottenthaler. P.O. Box 608, Camp Hill, Pa. 17011. (717) 763-7053.

171. PHILADELPHIA EMS FORUM. Philadelphia EMS Council, PHMC (Philadelphia Health Management Corp.), 530 Walnut Street, 13th Floor, Philadelphia, Pa. 19106. (215) 629-0575.

Sources

172. PITTSBURGH PARAMEDIC. Monthly. Ed. Roy E. Cox, Jr. Fraternal Association of Professional Paramedics, P.O. Box 10248, Pittsburgh, Pa. 15232. (412) 521-7339.

173. PRESIDENT'S NEWSLETTER. American Ambulance Association, 1401 Twenty-First Street, Sacramento, Calif. 95814. (916) 488-5223.

174. PULSE. 1975-- . Bimonthly. Official Journal of the American Association of Trauma Specialists, 3528 North Ashland Avenue, Chicago, Ill. 60657. (312) 263-0800.

175. REGISTRY EMT NEWSLETTER. Quarterly. National Registry of EMTs, 1395 East Granville Road, P.O. Box 29233, Columbus, Ohio 43229. (614) 888-4484.

176. RESPONDER. 10 per year. Ed. Vicki Smith. East Central Florida EMS Council, 1008 North Orlando Avenue, Winter Park, Fla. 32789. (305) 644-6911.

177. RESPONSE EMS ALASKA. 1978-- . Bimonthly. Ed. Gloria Houston. Alaska Section of EMS, Pouch H-06C, Juneau, Alaska 99811. (907) 465-3027.

178. RESPONSE TIME. Quarterly. Ed. Evelyn Beasch. North Dakota Association of EMTs, Lisbon, N.D. 58054. (701) 683-5946.

179. SIREN. 1947-- . Monthly. Ed. Barbara Ethridge. California Ambulance Association, P.O. Box 28709, Sacramento, Calif. 95828. (916) 443-5959.

180. SOUTH CAROLINA RESCUE NEWS. 1967-- . Bimonthly. South Carolina Association of Rescue Squads, P.O. Box 426, Barnwell, S.C. 29812.

181. STAT. Delaware County Emergency Health Services Council, Media Courthouse, Media, Pa. 19063. (215) 891-2676.

182. TEMTA NEWS. Monthly. Ed. Robert Brooks. Tennessee EMT Association, P.O. Box 4648, Nashville, Tenn. 37216. (615) 331-6225.

183. TEXAS EMERGENCY MEDICAL SERVICES MESSENGER. 1975-- . Quarterly. Texas State Department of Health, Emergency Medical Services Division, 1100 West Forty-Ninth Street, Austin, Tex. 78756.

184. TRAUMA CENTER NEWSLETTER. 1970-- . Monthly. Department of Surgery. Abraham Lincoln School of Medicine, P.O. Box 6998, Chicago, Ill. 60680.

185. TRAUMAGRAM. 1974-- . Quarterly. American Trauma Society, 875 North Michigan Avenue, Chicago, Ill. 60611. (312) 649-1810.

Sources

186. TRAUMA LINE. 1971-- . Quarterly. Ed. Charles N. Perry. Maryland State Ambulance and Rescue Association, 2405 Tionesta Road, Lansdowne, Baltimore, Md. 21227. (301) 242-5112.

187. UNSCHEDULED EVENTS. Disaster Research Center. Ohio State University, 127-129 West Tenth Avenue, Columbus, Ohio 43201.

188. VOICE OF MRFAA. Monthly. Ed. John Rukavina. Minnesota Rescue and First Aid Association, 1836 West Shryer Avenue, Roseville, Minn. 55113. (612) 376-3535.

189. WEST ALABAMA EMERGENCY MEDICAL SERVICES. Bimonthly. P.O. Box 911, University, Ala. 35386. (205) 345-0938.

190. WESTCHESTER COUNTY EMS NEWSLETTER. Bimonthly. Ed. Wallace Owen. Valhalla, N.Y. 10595. (914) 347-7244.

191. WINDS. Monthly. Ed. Jim Murray. Wyoming Ambulance and Emergency Medical Services Association, Cheyenne, Wyo. 82002. (307) 777-7955.

E. AUDIOVISUAL AIDS

The field of EMS audiovisuals is a large one. EMS audiovisuals cover both the clinical and the systems aspects. Only the systems aspect will be dealt with in this guide. The free market spirit of the United States was spurred by the influx of monies coming from federal sources, mainly through the EMSS Act of 1973 and amendments. This created a flood of audiovisuals of marginal quality and usefulness. Hundreds, maybe even thousands, of individuals and organizations devoted themselves to the creation of audiovisuals of some possible use in EMS education.

To recommend a certain item in this field is dangerous. The best way to select an audiovisual item is to preview it, and, keeping in mind the particular needs and objectives of the program in question, decide if the audiovisual is relevant or not.

These organizations can provide information--where to find what--on films, cassettes, and similar media available for loan and/or purchase.

Some main sources for audiovisuals are:

192. Academy of Health Sciences, U.S. Army, Fort Sam Houston, Tex. 78234. (512) 221-1211.

193. American Heart Association Film Library, Distribution Department, 44 East Twenty-Third Street, New York, N.Y. 10010. (212) 661-5335.

194. American Hospital Association Film Library, 840 North Lake Shore Drive, Chicago, Ill. 60611. (312) 645-9400.

Sources

195. American Medical Association Film Library, 525 North Dearborn Street, Chicago, Ill. 60610 (312) 715-6000.

196. Emergency Care Information Center, 701 Ridgefield Road, Wilton, Conn. 06897. (203) 762-3911.

197. Emergency Medical Services Information Center, American College of Emergency Physicians, 3900 Capital City Boulevard, Lansing, Mich. 48906. (517) 321-7911.

198. Fernández-Caballero, Carlos, and Otterbein, Scott A. Emergency Medical Services Audiovisuals. Rev. ed. Philadelphia: Center for the Study of Emergency Health Services, 1975. 199 p.

199. National Audiovisual Center (GSA), Washington, D.C. 20409.

Chapter 3
EMERGENCY MEDICAL SERVICES ORGANIZATIONS

A. ORGANIZATIONS—DIRECT INVOLVEMENT WITH EMS

Direct involvement is understood as an organization whose main activities are directed toward the different aspects of EMS.

200. ACT Foundation
(Advanced Coronary Treatment)
Basking Ridge, N.J. 07920
(201) 766-2273

201. Ambulance and Medical Services Association (AMSA)
Founded 1974
P.O. Box 14178
Hartford, Conn. 06114

202. American Academy of Orthopaedic Surgeons, Founded 1933
(Committee on Injuries, founded 1962)
430 North Michigan Avenue
Chicago, Ill. 60611
(312) 822-0970

203. American Ambulance Association
1919 Market Street
Youngstown, Ohio 44507
(216) 755-2111

204. American Association for the Surgery of Trauma
Founded 1938
University of Colorado Medical Center
Denver, Colo. 80220
(303) 394-8718

205. American Association of Critical Care Nurses
Founded 1969
P.O. Box 19528
Irvine, Calif. 92713
(714) 752-8191

206. American Association of Trauma Specialists
1052 North Northwest Highway
Park Ridge, Ill. 60068
(312) 692-5750

207. American Association of Trauma Specialists Education Foundation
1052 North Northwest Highway
Park Ridge, Ill. 60068
(312) 692-5750

208. American Board of Emergency Medicine
3900 Capital City Boulevard
Lansing, Mich. 48906
(517) 321-7911

209. American Burn Association
New York Hospital-Cornell Medical Center
525 East Sixty-Eighth Street, Room F-758
New York, N.Y. 10021

Organizations

210. American College of Emergency Physicians, Chartered 1968
3900 Capital City Boulevard
Lansing, Mich. 48906
(517) 321-7911

211. American College of Surgeons
Founded 1913
(Committee on Injuries, founded 1962)
55 East Erie Street
Chicago, Ill. 60611
(312) 664-4050

212. American Trauma Society
Founded 1971
875 North Michigan Avenue, Suite 3010
Chicago, Ill. 60611
(312) 649-1810

213. Burn Foundation of Greater Delaware Valley
250 South Seventeenth Street
Philadelphia, Pa. 19103

214. Emergency Care Research Institute, founded 1965
5200 Butler Pike
Plymouth Meeting, Pa. 19462
(215) 825-6000

215. Emergency Department Nurses Association, founded 1970
666 North Lake Shore Drive
Chicago, Ill. 60611
(312) 649-0297

216. Emergency Medical Services Administrators Association
Founded 1974
P.O. Box 43
EDM Station
Des Moines, Iowa 50309

217. Emergency Medical Services Education Association
P.O. Box 5346
Tacoma, Wash. 98405

218. Emergency Medicine Foundation
3900 Capital City Boulevard
Lansing, Mich. 48906
(517) 321-7911

219. Emergency Medicine Residents Association
3900 Capital City Boulevard
Lansing, Mich. 48906
(517) 321-7031

220. EMT Apprenticeship Program, IAFC/IAFF
1750 New York Avenue, N.W.
Washington, D.C. 20006
(202) 833-2274

221. International Rescue and First Aid Association
3200 Valleyview Drive
Columbus, Ohio 43204
(614) 274-7750

222. Interphase EMS Foundation
P.O. Box 2205
Calgary, Alberta, Canada
T2P 2M7
(403) 283-6868

223. National Association of Emergency Medical Technicians
P.O. Box 334
Newton Highlands, Mass. 02161
(617) 894-7179

224. National Association of Emergency Paramedics
800 West Central Road
Arlington Heights, Ill. 60005
(312) 398-3875

225. National Registry of Emergency Medical Technicians, founded 1970
P.O. Box 29233
Columbus, Ohio 43229
(614) 888-4484

226. Society for Critical Care Medicine
Founded 1970
University of Pittsburgh
Pittsburgh, Pa. 15213
(412) 624-4141

227. Society of Teachers of Emergency Medicine
3900 Capital City Boulevard
Lansing, Mich. 48906
(517) 321-7698

Organizations

228. Society for Total Emergency
Programs (STEP)
214 Alexander Street
Rochester, N.Y. 14607
(716) 244-4460

229. University Association for EMS
3900 Capital City Boulevard
Lansing, Mich. 48906
(517) 321-7060

B. ORGANIZATIONS—PERIPHERAL INVOLVEMENT WITH EMS

Peripheral or indirect involvement refers to organizations which have a tangential interest in EMS.

230. American Heart Association
44 East Twenty-Third Street
New York, N.Y. 10010
(212) 477-9170

231. American Hospital Association
840 North Lake Shore Drive
Chicago, Ill. 60611
(312) 645-9400

232. American National Red Cross
Seventeenth and D Streets, N.W.
Washington, D.C. 20006
(202) 737-8300

233. American Public Health Association
Injury Control and Emergency
Health Services Section
1015 Eighteenth Street, N.W.
Washington, D.C. 20005
(202) 789-5600

234. Associated Public Safety Communication Officers
P.O. Box 669
New Smyrna Beach, Fla. 32069
(904) 427-3461

235. Public Safety Officers Foundation
307 North Michigan Avenue,
Suite 2024
Chicago, Ill. 60601

C. GOVERNMENTAL AND OFFICIAL (OR SEMIOFFICIAL AGENCIES)

236. Federal Communications Commission
1919 M Street, N.W.
Washington, D.C. 20054

237. National Research Council–
National Academy of Sciences
Division of Medical Sciences
Committee on Trauma; Committee on Shock
2101 Constitution Avenue, N.W.
Washington, D.C. 20418

238. Office of Telecommunication Policy
1800 G Street, N.W.
Washington, D.C. 20504

239. U.S. Department of Health and Human Services
Division of Emergency Medical Services
6525 Belcrest Road
West Hyattsville, Md. 20782

240. U.S. Department of Transportation
National Highway Traffic Safety
Administration, Rescue and Emergency Medical Services Division
400 Seventh Street, N.W.
Washington, D.C. 20590

Chapter 4
LITERATURE

A. MANPOWER AND TRAINING

PL 93-154, the EMSS Act of 1973, lists a set of fifteen requirements.[3] The first two requirements are manpower and personnel training.

Manpower refers to the staffing of an EMSS by an adequate number of employees to cover services twenty-four hours a day, seven days a week. Some of the personnel required are: (1) first responders: fire, police, and other safety people; (2) communication personnel; (3) EMT-As, and EMT-Ps; (4) nurses; (5) administrators at all levels, and (6) physicians.

Training: Adequate training, and continuing education must be provided for the professionals enumerated under manpower. This training must be regionally coordinated. The law also recommends the recruitment and training of veterans of the Armed Forces with experience in health care fields.

These two components are presented here together because, for all practical purposes, both are closely intertwined.

241. Alongi, Sharon, et al. "Physician and Patient Acceptance of Emergency Nurse Practitioners." JACEP 8 (September 1979): 357-59.

> Patient and physician attitudes toward emergency nurse practitioners were surveyed in our emergency medical service. The response to the questionnaires indicated a high degree of satisfaction with the ENP similar to that reported in a survey of patient reaction to physician assistants in the emergency department. (Author's Abstract)

242. American College of Emergency Physicians. <u>A Guide for a Workshop to Identify the Physician as the Key Figure for Improving Emergency Medical Services in the Community.</u> East Lansing, Mich.: 1972. 24 p.

---

3. The description of all fifteen components is based on: <u>The EMSS Act of 1973</u> and <u>EMSS Program Guidelines, 1979.</u>

Literature

ACEP initiated this plan for a workshop to demonstrate that the physician has the key role in developing and improving emergency medical services. Chapter headings are as follows: "Leadership"; "Gather Information to Determine the Extent of Need"; "Seek out allies"; "Implementation of Program"; "Maintain Program on Continuing Basis"; and "Key to Public Support."

243. American Medical Association. <u>Guide to Program Planning</u>: <u>Emergency Medical Service Technician.</u> Chicago: 1972. 33 p.

    This guide, prepared by the AMA and the American Association of Junior Colleges, outlines a four-semester junior college program for the training of emergency medical technicians (EMTs). Some of the major topics covered are: the role of the EMT; his/her skills and treatment; and legal considerations.

244. Anwar, Rebecca A.H. "Trends in Training: Focus on Emergency Medicine." <u>Annals of Emergency Medicine</u> 9 (February 1980): 60-71.

    This research project analyzes the development of emergency medicine residencies and compares it to surgical and internal medicine residencies. The following factors were studied: characteristics of the program founders, reasons why physicians chose to enter the program, program organizational and structural variations, and career patterns of physicians in the program.

245. Anwar, Rebecca A.H., and Hogan, Michael H. "Residency-Trained Physicians: Where Have All the Flowers Gone?" JACEP 8 (February 1979): 84-87.

    What will emergency physicians do after completing residency programs? Some critics of this new specialty claim that because emergency medicine has unique demands that are often stressful and undefined, most physicians will not remain long in the field. This question of the fate of emergency medicine residency graduates is central to research into the development of this new specialty.

246. Bennett, Margaret Jane. "The Social Worker's Role: The Social Service Department Can Contribute Materially to the Effectiveness of Care Rendered in the Emergency Department." <u>Hospitals</u> 47 (16 May 1973): 111, 114, 118.

    The social worker, with the support of the hospital administration and the emergency department staff, can contribute to the effectiveness of patient care rendered by the emergency department. The social worker is able to assist the patient, and his family during the patient's stay in the ED, and even after the emergency is over.

247. Block, Frank E., et al. "Self-Instructional Emergency Medicine Program for Medical Students." JACEP 6 (January 1977): 4-6.

Literature

A self-instructional program in emergency medicine has been developed for freshmen medical students at the University of Virginia School of Medicine. The cognitive objective of the course is to give the student the minimum level of knowledge to diagnose emergency medical conditions. As a result of successful completion of the training program, the student is certified as an EMT in the Commonwealth of Virginia.

248. Caldwell, Peggy. "Continuing Education for Emergency Nurses: California-Style." JEN 3 (July-August 1977): 27-32.

    The California Emergency Department Nurses Association presented the continuing education curriculum to its membership over a year ago. The curriculum consists of twenty-five modules outlining material an emergency nurse clinician ought to know. Its advantages are: (1) it gives some stability to the material presented under a given topic, and (2) it is aimed at emergency nursing, rather than "junior physicians."

249. Caroline, Nancy L. "Paramedic Training in the United States: The State of the Art." Para-Medical Journal (Fall 1975): 6-9.

    Training programs for EMT-paramedics vary in length from approximately one hundred to twelve hundred hours. The contents also vary. The author reviewed approximately thirty curricula. Available programs are described and a general philosophy for curriculum is suggested.

250. Cleven, Arlene. Emergency Medical Technician Instructor Training Institute. Darien, Conn.: Dunlap and Associates, June 1972. 175 p. (NTIS, PB-211/924)

    The purpose of the instructor-training institute was to familiarize state and local emergency medical instructional personnel with NHTSA-developed curriculum materials and to enhance their instructional capabilities with this material. A thirty-hour course was designed to correlate with the content of the EMT-ambulance course. Vocational education faculty of Central Connecticut State College were oriented to become EMT-ambulance teacher trainers. Five geographically dispersed institutions of higher education were selected as local hosts during the fall 1971. NHTSA, through its regional offices, state governor's representatives, and state or local agencies, identified and referred approximately thirteen trainees to each site.

251. Cronin, Kathie, et al. "First Aid and Emergency Care Training: Its Effect on Prehospital Emergency Care." JACEP 4 (July-August 1975): 309-12.

    The effect of first aid and the emergency care training program on the delivery of prehospital care was evaluated by screening 862 emergency department patients in a suburban Pittsburgh hospital. Results indicated that personnel who had

Literature

received the eighty-one hour EMT-ambulance course provided the most adequate prehospital care of emergency patients.

252. Dalen, James E., et al. "CPR Training for Physicians." New England Journal of Medicine 303 (21 August 1980): 455-57.

    The requirement that all physicians must demonstrate practical knowledge of cardiopulmonary resuscitation does not please all physicians. The authors put forward their belief that, in the best interest of physicians, and the public, all physicians must have formal training in CPR.

253. Eisenberg, Mickey S., et al. "Cardiac Resuscitation in the Community: Importance of Rapid Provision and Implications for Program Planning." JAMA 241 (4 May 1979): 1905-07.

    This paper studies several time-related variables involving resuscitation from out-of-hospital cardiac arrest. It is shown that 43 percent of victims survived if CPR begins within four minutes of collapse and if definitive care is initiated within eight minutes. Widespread CPR training of the populace is an important way to improve time of initiation of CPR. The instruction of emergency medical technicians in defibrillation techniques is an important way to improve time of provision of definitive care.

254. "Emergency Medicine: Alive and Well in L.A." Medical World News 14 (12 January 1973): 16-18.

    Los Angeles County-University of Southern California Medical Center has raised its emergency medical services to full-department status. Its EMT and physicians assistants training programs are described and it is emphasized that emergency medicine is a legitimate specialty which requires adequate and separate training.

255. Farrington, Joseph D. "EMT--A Registry Certifies Competence." JACEP 2 (March-April 1973): 111-12.

    While numerous standards and guidelines to assist in the improvement of EMS have been developed in the past six years, ambulance services lagged behind other health services in training and proficiency of personnel. The registry of EMTs was formed in 1970. Its purpose is to foster training and education of EMTs and to set and maintain standards for their training examinations leading to certification and national registration.

256. Fincke, Mildred K. "Emergency Nurse: Teacher and Leader." JEN 1 (January-February 1975): 25-26.

    The growing number of health personnel entering the field of emergency medicine is an exciting phenomenon in which nurses have played an important part. Emergency nursing provides a challenging and varied opportunity to extend nursing expertise. In many ways emergency nursing is unique, but it also shares much common ground with other nursing roles.

Literature

257. Flint, Lewis M., et al. "Development of Selection Criteria for Advanced EMT Trainees." JACEP 4 (November-December 1975): 536-38.

   The results of a standard psychological profile and test of awareness, in conjunction with biographical data and personal interviews, are used to select 21 persons from 142 candidates to attend an advanced EMT course. The data suggest that standard tests may be valuable adjuncts to biographical data and interviews for selection of students for advanced EMT training.

258. Fortuna, Joseph Amadeo. "Training the EHS Systems Administrator." Presented at the American Public Health Association Convention, New Orleans, 24 October 1974. 14 p.

   The paper outlines and identifies the need for adequately trained EMS administrators at different organizational levels. It also explains the development of a course to be offered in the future by the University of Pennsylvania Center for the Study of Emergency Health Services.

259. Frey, Charles F., and Mangold, Karl. "The Physician and the Emergency Health Service System." Postgraduate Medicine 55 (January 1974): 197-204.

   Few fully operational emergency health service systems exist today. Most systems are uncoordinated or deficient in at least one component. Efforts are under way at local, state, and national levels to improve transportation of the acutely ill or injured by training emergency care vehicle operators. The individual physician is working through professional organizations and emergency service councils to help develop area-wide planning of emergency health services.

260. Geolot, Denise, et al. "Emergency Nurse Practitioners: An Answer to an Emergency Care Crisis in Rural Hospitals." JACEP 6 (August 1977): 355-57.

   During the last three years, a nine-month training program at the University of Virginia was designed and implemented to prepare the nurse to assume an expanded role in the emergency department. The course provides the student with sufficient knowledge and skill to diagnose and treat patients in the emergency department setting while under the supervision of a physician.

261. Goldfrank, Lewis, et al. "The Emergency Services Physician Assistant: Results of Two Years' Experience." Annals of Emergency Medicine 9 (February 1980): 96-99.

   The physician assistant (PA) has become an integral part of urban health care. The roles chosen are diverse and often meet particular needs of physicians or hospitals. We have developed a unique program in emergency services that allows for training and development of PAs in two distinctly hospital settings. These PAs perform medical-surgical liaison work

Literature

bridging what, at times, can be a complex cultural gap. It is our premise that these individuals can significantly improve the quality and quantity of care rendered. (Authors' Abstract)

262. Grenvid, Ake. "Role of Allied Health Professionals in Critical Care Medicine." Critical Care Medicine 2 (January-February 1974): 6-10.

    The treatment of critically ill and injured patients in separate intensive care units has created a great need for a large number of paramedical specialists and technicians of various categories, among them: respiratory therapists, social workers, unit managers, bacteriologists, and emergency medical technicians. They can uniquely and significantly contribute to the improvement of intensive care as well as to the reduction of mortality and long-term invalidity.

263. Grigg, Thomas R., et al. "Impact of Medical Training on Ambulance Dispatching." JACEP 6 (February 1977): 47-49.

    This study was designed to assess the ability of trained individuals to screen calls for emergency medical services to allow for safer or more appropriate responses. The degree of urgency of calls, as judged by dispatchers and a panel of physicians, was compared to estimates of the severity of the patient's illness or injury. The EMTs were better able to assess severity and degree of urgency than were physicians or dispatchers.

264. Haeck, William T. "The Emerging Specialty of the Emergency Department Physician." Journal of the South Carolina Medical Association 69 (January 1973): 20-21.

    The emergency physician specialty was created in response to increased public demands on the emergency department. Two plans for staffing the emergency department with physicians at all times, the Alexandria Plan and the Pontiac Plan, were developed. The Pontaic Plan allows a large group of physicians to share responsibility for the emergency department; the Alexandria Plan requires physicians to limit their practice to the emergency department.

265. Hannas, Ralston R. "Emergency Department Physician Staffing Patterns and Residency Training." Illinois Medical Journal 143 (June 1973): 525-26.

    This article describes the Alexandria and Pontiac Plans for staffing emergency departments, and recommends the Residency Training Program in Emergency Medicine developed by the American College of Emergency Physicians in 1970.

266. Harrison, Robert R., and Maull, Kimball I. "Emergency Medical Technician (EMT-A) Instruction of Medical Students." JACEP 8 (December 1979): 513-14.

In 1977, the Department of Anesthesiology of the Medical College of Virginia coordinated a compulsory seventy-two hour course for first-year medical students fulfilling all requirements of the DOT and leading to eligibility for certification of the medical student as an EMT. This sound foundation in emergency care concepts enables the student to develop greater competence in critical skills during the clinical years.

267. Iserson, Kenneth V., and Shepherd, Clovis. "Teaching Emergency Department Administration: The In-Basket Exercise." JACEP 8 (March 1979): 114-15.

Borrowing from formats that have been used successfully in teaching administrators, a limited, time-dependent simulation model, the in-basket exercise, was developed for teaching emergency department administration. The exercise is designed as an introduction to nonclinical decisions, management communication, and managerial control. Using selected materials, and under time constraints, participants are asked to describe the options for several types of administrative problems.

268. Jayne, Harold A. "Modified Small Group ACLS Instructor/Provider Course." Annals of Emergency Medicine 9 (May 1980): 253-55.

This paper describes a method of combining instructor and provider advanced cardiac life support (ACLS) courses. This method overcomes both the problem of training and certifying a sufficient number of faculty and the difficulty of staffing an instructor-level course.

269. Kiefer, Joseph N. "Staffing and Other Problems of a Small Hospital Emergency Service." Master's thesis, Xavier University, 1976. 105 p.

This thesis examines some of the problems involved in providing emergency care, with emphasis on problems of the small hospital. The McCullough-Hyde Memorial Hospital, an eighty-one bed institution located in Oxford, Ohio, is assessed with regard to staffing, training, transportation, communications, costs, accreditation, and emergency medical services system. The author gives specific conclusions and recommendations.

270. Krome, Ronald, and Silva, Yvan J. "The Foreign Medical Grad on the Emergency Care Team." JACEP 1 (November-December 1972): 45-47.

Foreign medical graduates are an asset to hospitals in the United States, particularly in emergency departments. In their daily duties, however, it is imperative that they adapt to the American way of life without sacrificing their medical contributions.

271. Lambrew, Costas T. "The Paramedic: The Problem of Defining a Role." JEN 1 (July-August 1975): 15-16.

Literature

Paramedic is a term that needs to be more adequately defined. It is broadly used to refer to the allied health personnel who render advanced life support to ill or injured patients at the scene or en route to a hospital.

272. Ledger, Martha, and Cayten, C. Gene. "The EMS Administrator at School." Emergency Medical Services 5 (March–April 1976): 36-38, 40,42.

    The article briefly reviews the historical changes in emergency care delivery precipitating the need for educational support for EMS administrators. It discusses the development of two curricula and describes in detail four week-long intensive courses in planning, financing, implementation, and evaluation offered in 1975 by the Center for the Study of Emergency Health Services, University of Pennsylvania.

273. Lee, Sung R., and Klippel, Allen P. "Emergency Department Staffing to Improve Patient Management." JACEP 6 (February 1977): 53-55.

    The Emergency Department records at the St. Louis County Hospital were reviewed for 1973, 1974, and 1975. The distribution of patients was considered by the day of the week and hour of the day. The data showed that one third of patients had been seen by 2:36 P.M. and two thirds by 8:14 P.M. An analysis of peak patient load showed the first peak was around 11:00 A.M. and the second, a higher peak, around 7:00 P.M. More patients were seen on Tuesday and Saturday. This data can be used for an appropriate staffing pattern.

274. Levy, Richard, and Anwar, Rebecca A.H. "Orientation Program for Emergency Medicine Residents." JACEP 8 (February 1979): 77-80.

    An orientation curriculum was developed for incoming residents in emergency medicine at the University of Cincinnati in July 1976. The major objectives of the orientation were: (1) to identify and delineate the subject matter of emergency medicine; and (2) to review the basic elements of emergency medicine. Results of a pre- and post-test using the residency program at the Medical College of Pennsylvania (MCP) as a control group are presented.

275. Lowry, Jon W., and Lauro, Albert J. "A General EMS Curriculum for Residency Training." Annals of Emergency Medicine 9 (May 1980): 250-52.

    Based on the guidelines provided by the American College of Emergency Physicians, the Joint Commission on Accreditation of Hospitals, the Department of Health and Human Services, and program alumni, the authors looked into ways of improving the EMS curriculum for residency training of Charity Hospital of Louisiana at New Orleans.

276. Maatsch, Jack L., et al. "The Emergency Medicine Specialty Certification Examination (EMSCE)." JACEP 5 (July 1976): 529-34.

The article describes the historical development and general overview of the Emergency Medicine Board Examination.

277. MacCally, Michael, et al. "A Course in Emergency Care for First-Year Medical Students." JACEP 7 (January 1978): 720-23.

> A fifty-two hour course in emergency medicine for first-year medical students was developed from the DOT training program for EMTs. The objective was to train students to provide life support and emergency care in the field at the level of competence of the EMT.

278. McSwain, Charlene, et al. "The Use of a Criterion Performance Checklist to Improve Efficiency and Effectiveness in a CPR Self-Teaching Program." Journal of Medical Education 54 (September 1979): 736-38.

> A simple criterion performance checklist was developed from the AHAs standards which measured the management of obstructed airways for conscious and unconscious persons for one and two rescuers. The checklist was designed to help the students monitor their self-teaching and help instructors certify performance.

279. McSwain, Norman E., Jr. "Medical Control--What Is It?" JACEP 7 (March 1978): 114-16.

> Medical control is essentially divided into three phases: prospective, immediate, and retrospective. Adequate medical supervision of any paramedic system is necessary to guarantee quality of medical care. Anything short of physician control of pre-hospital medical care would be to abdicate our responsibilities to our patients. (Author's Abstract)

280. Mains, Kenneth D., et al. "A New Health Professional: The Trauma Coordinator." Illinois Medical Journal 142 (August 1972): 158-60.

> The (Illinois) trauma coordinator has many years of military training experience of casualty care and transportation and has become the mainstay of the Illinois Trauma Program. His basic responsibilities are: (1) data collection; (2) education; (3) communication and transportation; (4) biomedical equipment maintenance; and (5) community relations.

281. Mangold, Karl G. "Postgraduate Realities: Surviving in Emergency Medicine Practice." JACEP 7 (June 1978): 245-48.

> American College of Emergency Physicians (ACEP) members have written regarding recent contractual demands being made by some hospitals that may indicate that their boards and administrators are intruding upon the practice of medicine and profiting from professional fees generated by emergency physicians.

282. Mattson, Joel L., et al. "Advanced Casualty Care Training Using Animal Models." Military Medicine 145 (June 1980): 401-4.

Literature

In order that they be prepared to deliver emergency care during mass casualty crises, military medical personnel are being trained in lifesaving procedures, using animal models.

283. Mills, John, et al. "Effectiveness of Nurse Triage in the Emergency Department of an Urban County Hospital." JACEP 5 (November 1976): 877-82.

> The effectiveness of patient triage by a specially trained registered nurse in the emergency department of an urban county hospital, San Francisco General Hospital, was evaluated over a three-month period. Ambulatory patients thought to have nonemergent illnesses were directed to the walk-in service for physician evaluation and treatment; the remainder were seen in the emergency service. Error in triage was about equally divided between mistaken diagnosis and underestimated severity of illness. The overall accuracy of triage was 98 percent.

284. Morando, Rocco. "Emergency Medical Technician-Ambulance: Bringing Professional Care to the Victim." JEN 1 (July-August 1975): 13-14.

> Since 1970, there has been a widespread effort involving both lay and medical organizations to upgrade emergency medical ambulance services. The result is a trained EMT-ambulance whose exposure to a rigid course on prehospital emergency care has prepared him/her to respond to emergencies with a knowledge of immediate care for the critically ill or injured.

285. Myrick, Justin A., et al. "Emergency Medical Coordinators: First Responders for Rural Communities." Journal of the Medical Association of Georgia 68 (November 1979): 975-77.

> This is a report of a project which seeks to determine if first responders are a viable alternative to an ambulance service.

286. Page, James O. Effective Company Command for Company Officers in the Professional Fire Service. Alhambra, Calif.: Borden Pub., 1973. 160 p. Illus.

> The how-to book for supervisors of emergency personnel. This classic text aims at the sensitive issues of self-improvement, interpersonal relationships, and supervision. The book was written with the fire fighter in mind.

287. Pizzi, Walter F., et al. "Life-Support Training in High-Density Population Centers." Journal of Trauma 18 (November 1978): 777-80.

> The training of the nonmedical population in basic life-support skills may significantly reduce death and disability in medical emergencies. This is especially true in high-density urban areas where professional response time may be slowed by traffic. This paper discusses a pilot project in New York City which trained employees of twenty-four corporations to deal with medical-surgical emergencies.

Literature

288. Pratt, Franklin D., and McElroy, Charles R. "Undergraduate Medical Education: An Evaluation of First Aid and Emergency Medicine Components." JACEP 7 (December 1978): 429-33.

    A questionnaire was mailed to 114 American medical schools to determine how and when students are taught components of first aid and emergency medicine, as well as the relationship between emergency medicine studies and those of traditional specialties. Only one of the 44 responding schools did not have an emergency facility available to students.

289. Romano, Teresa L. "Emergency Nurse Education: The Emergency Physician." JACEP 7 (January 1978): 27-28.

    Emergency department nurses are the greatest untapped resource in the ranks of emergency medical services (EMS) personnel. Although in many rural hospitals they are often the first, and sometimes the only person to see a patient, no aggressive attempts have been made to update their definitive care capability or their level of responsibility.

290. _____. "The Future of Nursing in Emergency Care." JEN 1 (January-February 1975): 19-21.

    Nurses need to be active members of the emergency team. They need to be trusted with more responsibilities and adequate training.

291. _____. "Trauma Nursing in Illinois." Hospitals 47 (16 May 1973): 147, 150-54.

    Although the physician remains the leader of the trauma team, the trauma nurse specialists are capable of exercising their clinical judgment and skills independently. Trauma nurse specialists are trained at six regional trauma centers to evaluate emergency patients, make diagnoses, and initiate appropriate treatment.

292. _____, et al. "Paramedic Services: Nationwide Distribution and Management Structure." JACEP 7 (March 1978): 99-102.

    A paramedic clearinghouse to provide information on the status of advanced life support systems in the United States is being established at the Center for the Study of Emergency Health Services, University of Pennsylvania, Philadelphia.

293. Scott, John E. "NIH and EMS Residency Training Programs." JACEP 1 (November-December 1972): 49-51.

    While several associations and institutions are interested in establishing new residencies and specialty boards in emergency medicine, the author points out that existing training programs in public health and preventive medicine are adequate for the training of an emergency management specialist.

Literature

294. Shabazian, Dawn. "Mobile Intensive Care Unit Nurse." JEN 1 (July-August 1975): 20-22.

    The author narrates her daily experiences at the communication center of the Little Company of Mary Hospital, Torrance, California.

295. Silverston, Paul P. "A Decade on the Road." Nursing Mirror 150 (March 1980): 16-18.

    The author describes the requisites and the training that a nurse needs in order to become an active member of a mobile intensive care unit.

296. Skelton, Mary Beth, and McSwain, Norman E. "A Study of Cognitive and Technical Skill Deterioration Among Trained Paramedics." JACEP 6 (October 1977): 436-38.

    Thirty trained paramedics were studied to measure cognitive and technical skill deterioration six to thirty months after completion of their individual training programs. The purpose of the study was to identify areas in need of continuing education and to see if the new rate of skill deterioration correlated with the time from completion of the training program. Skills requiring the most technical knowledge deteriorated the fastest.

297. Smith, Leslie R. "From Ambulance Driver to EMT." Hospitals 47 (16 May 1973): 105-8.

    In 1968, the National Academy of Sciences analyzed regulations for ambulance personnel training throughout the nation and found that seventy different programs using twenty different textbooks existed. There were no generally accepted standards of proficiency. In a contract report to the U.S. Department of Transportation, Dunlap Associates stressed the need for well-trained EMTs. Dunlap subsequently developed a course and selected a single textbook.

298. Sourwine, R.E. "'E' Squads are Prepared to Respond to any Kind of Crisis Situation." Occupational Health Safety 47 (May-June 1978): 48-50.

    The training techniques to prepare workers and guards of the Chemical Division of PPG Industries, Pittsburgh, Pennsylvania, to handle emergencies is described.

299. Spitz, Louis, et al. "Psychiatric Training for Emergency Medicine Residents on a Multidisciplinary Team." JACEP 5 (September 1976): 694-97.

    The Cincinnati General Hospital Emergency Department has a training program for emergency medicine residents on a multidisciplinary emergency psychiatry team. This training should occur in the ED setting rather than in psychiatric inpatient units of state hospital settings. Nonmedical members of the emergency psychiatric team train and support emergency medicine residents in a multidisciplinary approach to treatment.

Literature

300. Stafford, Valerie G. "The Emergency Nurse Practitioner: The Role and Training of an Emerging Health Professional." JACEP 7 (October 1978): 372-76.

   In recent years, the roles of various health care professionals have changed to better provide health services to the consumer. This work describes the inception, training, and role of the nurse practitioner, compares the nurse practitioner to the physician's assistant and physician surrogate, and examines the need for and role of the emergency department nurse practitioner.

301. "Standards and Guidelines for Cardiopulmonary Resuscitation (CPR) and Emergency Cardiac Care (ECC)." JAMA 244 (1 August 1980): 453-509.

   These standards and guidelines encompass: (1) principles and techniques for the performance of basic and advanced cardiac life support; (2) standards for training and certification in basic life support as defined by the American Heart Association; (3) recommendations for training, testing, and supervision of medical and allied health personnel; (4) the proposed role of the American Red Cross and other agencies in the training of the lay public; (5) a renewed, strong emphasis on community acceptance of responsibllity for coronary heart disease morbidity and mortality and acceptance of organized implementation of primary and secondary prevention programs in parallel with ECC efforts; (6) definition of the role of ECC units in stratified systems of emergency care; and (7) medicolegal aspects of CPR and ECC. (Publication's Abstract)

302. Staroscik, Rudolf, and Cayten, C. Gene. "Emergency Medical Technician-Paramedic Training." JACEP 5 (August 1976): 605-8.

   With a nationally standardized EMT-paramedic training program soon to be adopted, certain factors in the planning of training programs should be emphasized: (1) the facilities should provide an opportunity for the paramedics to gain clinical experience; (2) the course content should include advanced life-support; (3) full-time and part-time programs must be developed; (4) the operating procedure should conform to local medical and legal practice; (5) mechanisms for evaluation and recertification must be developed; and (6) continuing education should be included in program planning.

303. Taubenhaus, Leon J. "Community Education for Emergency Services." JACEP 2 (January-February 1973): 36-38.

   EMS form a four-phase spectrum which include the emergency itself, emergency transportation, ED care, and follow-up care. A program expanding the role of the emergency physician is in progress under a community health service. To improve care in phase 1, ten ten-hour courses have been given to a total of 810 laymen. Bilingual courses for local residents and courses for nearby occupational health personnel are contemplated. A forty-five hour program is offered to ambulance personnel.

Literature

304. _____. "The Training of House Officers in the Emergency Department." JACEP 6 (November-December 1973): 401-4.

    The training of residents and interns in the ED has been largely a hit-or-miss matter in most teaching hospitals, according to the results of a study conducted among 467 university-affiliated hospitals. Of the 118 institutions which responded to the questionnaire, there was little commonality of training programs for house staff in the ED. Most interns and residents enter the ED with little medical school training in the field and find, in the majority of cases, a poorly organized training experience.

305. Taylor, Dianne P. The Utilization of a Psychiatric Nurse by the Staff of an Emergency Room: A Replication. New Haven, Conn.: Yale University, 1977. 90 p.

    This study of the use of a psychiatric nurse clinician in the ED was a replication of a 1971 study. Of the fifty-four situations studied, nineteen were psychiatrically oriented, and thirty-five were nonpsychiatrically oriented. The staff formally requested the nurse intervention in twenty-two situations, while she informally initiated her own involvement in thirty-two situations. The results indicate that the need for a psychiatric nurse clinician in the ED has decreased in the five years since the original study.

306. Tye, J.B., et al. "Survey of Continuing Education Needs for Non-Emergency Physicians in Emergency Medicine." JACEP 7 (January 1978): 16-19.

    A questionnaire was mailed to every physician in Iowa (2,551) to determine their need for continuing education in emergency medicine. Results revealed a low incidence of formal education in emergency medicine, particularly at the undergraduate and graduate levels. The primary conclusion of the study is that continued education in basic emergency medical care is perceived as being necessary for physicians who are not specialists in emergency medicine.

307. Waekerle, Joseph F., et al. "The Emergency Nurse as a Primary Health Care Provider: A Retrospective Study." JEN 3 (July-August 1977): 21-26.

    This article describes the historical development of the role and function of the emergency nurse. There is emphasis on the work performed by the nurse practitioner and how that experience can be applied to the emergency department triage situation.

308. Watkins, Richard N., et al. "Educational Audit: One Department's Approach in an HMO Setting." JACEP 6 (April 1977): 147-54.

    The emergency staff of a large prepaid group practice developed a system of in-house education for practicing emergency physicians based directly on feedback from their own practice.

Literature

This feedback is derived from: (1) the continuous audit of cases suggested for review by colleagues, and (2) intermittent audit in the conventional manner of selected clinical entities. The theory of this system is that physician's education should be based on individual strengths and weaknesses identified by the audit.

309. Weiner, Mary Anne, et al. "Inservice Training for Rural Nurses in Emergency Care Concepts and Skills." JEN 1 (March-April 1975): 16-23.

    A thirty-hour in-service training program in emergency care concepts and skills was developed and held for rural nurses with major emphasis on giving nurses experience and confidence in carrying out basic but crucial lifesaving procedures while the physician is still en route to the emergency department.

310. White, Roger D. "Physician's Role in Ambulance Service." JACEP 1 (November-December 1972): 39-42.

    Physicians are the most important element in the training of emergency medical technicians (EMT) and must participate actively in this service. Only in this manner can deficient ambulance service throughout the country be improved.

311. Witt, Richard C., and Haedtler, David R. "Nurse-Scribe System Saves Time in the E.D." JEN 1 (January-February 1975): 22-24.

    Emergency departments throughout the country are finding they can save valuable time while providing comprehensive emergency treatment by using a nurse-scribe and physician team as the central moving force. A nurse-scribe is a nurse who works as the physician's right arm by recording notes on the patient's chart as ordered by the physician, then implementing the appropriate treatment under the physician's direction.

B. COMMUNICATIONS

This section posits the joining of personnel, facilities, and equipment by a central communications system, which will facilitate the telephonic screening of emergency calls. The system might, or might not, implant the universal emergency telephone number 911.

The brain and heart of this section is the resource management center through its central dispatch function.

312. Allenbaugh, Gerald E. "Radios Restore Order to Chaos." Hospitals 46 (16 January 1972): 60-65.

    The experience of the Los Angeles earthquake of 9 February 1971 demonstrated that a well-organized communication network was essential to the implementation of disaster plans. This

Literature

paper describes how well-trained hospital personnel, through the emergency radio network, provided fast and coordinated response during the critical hours after the disaster. A history and disaster plan for the Los Angeles area is also provided.

313. Beaman, Wrex W., et al. <u>Communications Plan for Emergency Medical Systems.</u> San Francisco: Bay Area Comprehensive Health Planning Council, November 1974. 22 p.

    Details of a radio communications plan for the Emergency Medical Services (EMS) system of the nine-county San Francisco Bay area are presented. The role of the Federal Communication Commission in authorizing eight channels for direct emergency care is discussed, including the use of biomedical telemetry on certain channels. The geographical features of the area present some difficulty in two-way radio coverage, and the suggestion is made that base stations should use existing high elevation transmitting sites as they are more efficient and economical.

314. Bouzarth, William F., and Mariano, John P. "Hospitals Emergency Code Systems: Study of a Communication Problem." JACEP 2 (January-February 1973): 33-35.

    A survey of seventy-five hospitals in the Philadelphia Standard Metropolitan Statistical Area (Philadelphia, Bucks, Chester, Delaware, and Montgomery counties) was conducted to select the system of communicating emergencies. Recommendations for standardization include use of discriminatory one-digit or low numerical, repetitive digit telephone numbers followed by the location of the life-threatening emergency.

315. Comprehensive Health Planning Council of South Florida. <u>Objectives of EMS Communications System.</u> Miami: April 1973. 9 p.

    Communication needs of the emergency medical service (EMS) system in Dade County, Florida, are outlined. Five basic communication needs are identified: (1) medical rescue-physician consultation, coordination, ambulances, and back up assistance; (2) medical facilities--interhospital and intra-hospital coordination and hospital (physician) to field communication procedures; (3) ambulance service--notification and dispatching procedures and links to medical facilities; (4) disasters--resource gathering and resource coordination; and (5) public access. Links among various EMS communications system components are noted and illustrated in a flow chart.

316. Drury, Colin G., and Schiro, Samuel George. "Evaluation of an EMS Communications System." JACEP 6 (April 1977): 133-38.

    This article reports the evaluation of a medical emergency radio system in Erie County, New York. It emphasizes the evaluation of problems in human-machine interface and the use of radio data by hospitals. The system was generally reliable and effective, but changes in organization and training could enhance the quality and usefulness of the system.

Literature

317. Garret, C.W. "MIEMS, Part 2: The Maryland Emergency Medical Services Communications System." <u>Maryland State Medical Journal</u> 27 (June 1978): 53-58.

> The construction of the Maryland Emergency Medical Services Communications System is described. In 1978, Maryland had the first complete EMS Communications system in the nation.

318. Grundy, Betty L., et al. "Telemedicine in Critical Care: An Experiment in Health Care Delivery." JACEP 6 (October 1977): 439-44.

> This experiment in telemedicine developed the following conclusions: (1) regular consultations in critical care can be provided by audiovisual link; (2) current technology is adequate but expensive; (3) telemedicine consultations can be made acceptable to users and providers; (4) telemedicine can be a valuable educational resource; (5) telemedicine can influence the process and probably the outcome of patient care; (6) the audiovisual link is superior to telephone for these consultations; and (7) telemedicine can serve as an important link between a small hospital and a large medical center, improving in that way the quality of care in the emergency unit of the small hospital.

319. Gustafson, Gerald E. "Radio, Training Spur Improvement." <u>Hospitals</u> 47 (May 1973): 131-34.

> The implementation of Tulsa's emergency medical communications system is described. The radio network, which allows two-way communications between ambulances and hospitals, was financed by physicians, hospitals, and donations from groups and individuals. The development of an EMT course is also discussed.

320. Henry, William J. "Alternative to 911." <u>Emergency Medicine Today</u> 3 (September 1974): 1-4.

> This article presents an alternative to the 911 system which was implemented in Methow Valley, north central Washington. A private number was established and five telephones were installed answering this number. They were located in the medical center, in the home of a physician, in the home of a trauma-trained nurse and in the homes of two ambulance drivers. Lists of on-duty personnel are posted beside each phone along with the number of the fire and police units.

321. Jarmon, Robert G. "Cardiac Telemetry Exercise Program." JACEP 6 (February 1977): 50-52.

> A program to train cardiac consultants was designed to evaluate electrocardiogram rhythm strips from the field. It was prepared as a series of prerecorded telemetered rhythms and discussions which could be sent into telemetry consoles. The consultant is requested to interpret the data and give advice to the EMT. At the end of the exercise, the student performance is evaluated.

Literature

322. Keller, Geraldine B. <u>Messages Received at an EMS Dispatching Center: Study of the Nature and Effect.</u> Columbus: Ohio State University Research Foundation, December 1976. 12 p.

    When a telephone call comes to the central emergency medical dispatch unit in Columbus, Ohio, the dispatcher could make one of the following decisions: (1) to send a standard ambulance; (2) to send a mobile coronary care unit (MCCU); or (3) to send no vehicle at all. Similar evaluation is made of the decision by the vehicle personnel to transport or not to the hospital, and the decision at the hospital to admit or not to admit for care.

323. Lambrew, Costas T., et al. "Emergency Medical Transport Systems: Use of ECG Telemetry." <u>Chest</u> 63 (April 1973): 477-82.

    This article describes a rapid response, widely deployed emergency medical transport system utilizing trained non-professional personnel supervised and evaluated by physicians through a patient communications system incorporating ECG telemetry. This has been developed within the framework of existing resources at relatively low cost. Analysis of the course and of the telemetered ECG of one thousand patients indicates that clinical deterioration, death, as well as life threatening arrhythmias occur in a significant number of patients en route to the hospital. These occurrences are not confined to patients with acute myocardial infarction. Such a system is feasible and justified to reduce prehospital morbidity and mortality in patients with acute illness or injury through arrhythmia control and cardiopulmonary resuscitation.

324. McDermott, Steve. "Planning for EMS Communications: A Review of Objectives to be Met in Implementing an EMS Communication System." <u>Emergency Medical Services</u> 2 (November-December 1973): 34-37.

    Effective communications planning is the most neglected component of EMS, one which is lacking in many model EMS systems. Problems in implementing EMS communications do not stem from lack of technology, but rather from inadequate planning and setting of objectives. The objectives delineated for EMS communications in Dade County, Florida, are presented. The components of the EMS system are discussed in terms of what they require of a communication system.

325. Murphy, Raymond L.H., and Bird, Kenneth T. "Telediagnosis: A New Community Health Resource." <u>American Journal of Public Health</u> 64 (February 1974): 113-19.

    This article reports on a program which demonstrates that telemedicine can increase the availability of quality medical care by means of a two-way audiovisual microwave circuit. Physicians at the Massachusetts General Hospital provided medical care to patients at the Logan International Airport Medical Station, almost three miles away.

Literature

326. Nagel, Eugene I. Telemetry and Physician-Rescue Personnel Communications. Miami: University of Miami, School of Medicine, September 1971. 204p. (NTIS, PB-206-298)

   This demonstration project tested the feasibility of advanced emergency medical care supplied by paramedical personnel. Advanced modalities included defibrillation, intravenous fluids and drugs, and telemetered electrocardiographic and voice communication with medical personnel in the hospital. Communications included base station (hospital) and mobile physician interchange with paramedics. Advanced training programs for fire rescue were designed and tested. Community response (medical and lay) was tested as to acceptance of these treatment modalities. Comparisons were made of resultant system and other test systems. Evaluation was made of ability of the system to respond quickly to all types of medical emergencies, special applicability to highway accident victims (traumatic and natural disease), and estimates made of system effectiveness if extended over large population areas.

327. _____, et al. "Telemetry-Medical Command in Coronary and Other Mobile Emergency Care Systems." JAMA 214 (12 October 1970): 332-38.

   A total of 146 victims were monitored by means of a telemetry medical system. This program was operated by in-hospital emergency physicians and rescue personnel. This system offers advantages over new and special physician staffed systems in that it has very fast response times and uses highly trained EMT-paramedics. Also, it possesses immediate availability at lower cost, and permits higher utilization.

328. National Highway Traffic Safety Administration (DOT). Communications Guidelines for Emergency Medical Services. Washington, D.C.: September 1972. 73 p. (DOT-HS-820-214)

   Information and guidance are provided for persons involved in planning and implementing emergency medical communications systems. The purpose of such systems is to reduce morbidity and mortality by bringing injured persons and definitive medical care together in the shortest possible time. Types of emergency medical systems (EMS) communications systems include: universal emergency telephone number; other telephone systems; phone and radio patch; paying systems; selective calling methods; physiological monitoring telemetry; and medical facilities data banks. It is noted that Federal Communications Commission regulations form a boundary to the EMS communications plan. The commission's rules involve frequency availability, applicant eligibility, and permissible communications rules. Suggestions are offered for implementing the EMS communications system, and sample data sheets are provided for a community EMS survey. A model of an EMS communication system is provided.

Literature

329. _____. Dispatcher Emergency Medical Technician Training Course. Washington, D.C.: 1972. 27 p.

> This instructor's guide to use of emergency communications systems contains seven lessons on ambulance dispatching, telephone techniques, voice techniques, and use of the radiotelephone at a base station or in a mobile unit, law enforcement and defense civil preparedness communications, equipment, and a sample testing procedure. The course serves as an adjunct to the Department of Transportation's Basic Training Program for Emergency Medical Technicians-Ambulance.

330. National Maritime Research Center. Feasibility Study for the Development and Use of the Satellite Communications System to Provide Shipboard Emergency Medical Services. Kings Point, N.Y.: April 1976. 70 p.

> This study investigates the current state of the art of shipboard medical care and develops a program for the feasibility of utilizing the MarAd Satellite Navigation-Communication System for medical emergency service of merchant seamen while at sea.

331. Office of Telecommunications Policy. Emergency Telephone Number (911). A Handbook for Community Planning. Washington, D.C.: Government Printing Office, May 1973. 70 p.

> A handbook for use by communities in planning for, installing and operating 911 emergency telephone number systems is presented. The booklet describes the history of 911; the potential benefits of the system with regard to crime rate, accident fatality, and fire losses; related policy statements, legislation, and endorsements; planning considerations; installation considerations; methods of operations; and costs likely to be involved. 911 is intended as a nationwide telephone number giving the public direct access to an emergency answering center.

332. Penterman, Daniel G. "A Case Study in Telecommunications." Emergency Medical Services 3 (May-June 1974): 16-19.

> The author comments on Nebraska's effort to provide for statewide EMS communications from 1965 on. Nebraska Legislative Act of 1967 established the State Telecommunications Bureau and recognized the importance of emergency communications. Since 1967, Nebraska has shown that with proper direction it is possible to organize overgrown systems and radio frequency clutter into an efficient communications system.

333. Sandifer, Calvin R. "A Study to Evaluate the Existing Emergency Medical Services Communications Network and Determine the Requirements for an Integrated Emergency Medical Services Communications System for the Shreveport-Bossier City, Louisiana Metropolitan Area." Master's thesis, Baylor University, Waco, Texas, August 1975. 80 p.

Literature

A two-week evaluation of the emergency medical services (EMS) and public safety communications network of the Shreveport-Bossier City, Louisiana, Metropolitan Area was conducted in March 1974 to determine the requirements for a viable communications system for the area. The system, as a minimum, had to be compatible with existing independent medical and public safety communications systems and serve as the core system for the ten-parish Northwest Louisiana Health Planning Region. It was concluded that an optimum communications system, which meets federal and private subsidy requirements, can be implemented only in conjunction with a local emergency operations center which includes a telephone switchboard terminal for a common, community-wide emergency telephone number.

334. Siler, Kenneth F. "Predicting Demand for Public Dispatched Ambulances in a Metropolitan Area." Health Services Research Management 10 (1975): 254-63.

A model is described for predicting ambulance demand, based on data from Los Angeles County ambulance systems. An estimated 2.4 million visits were made between June 1973 and June 1974 to approximately 190 emergency facilities in Los Angeles County. Application of the model showed that the demand for public emergency vehicles appears to be highly predictable using a nonlinear per capita formula employing socioeconomic land use, and emergency medical services parameters.

335. Smalley, Harold E. Telemetry Utilization for Emergency Medical Services System. Atlanta: Georgia Institute of Technology, June 1974. 76 p. (NTIS PB-242/082)

This work is a guide for emergency medical services planners to assist them in the determination of the feasibility of telemetry utilization in their own EMS system. This report also can serve as an aid in designing new EMS systems, and employs information furnished by the user to determine the desirability, possibility, and necessity of using telemetry in order to achieve an effective level of emergency coronary care.

336. Southern Maine Comprehensive Health Association. Southern Maine's Emergency Medical Communication System. Portland: April 1973. 38 p.

Terms and definitions are provided, and operating instructions are given for the regional hospitals, including diagrams of the General Electric and Motorola control consoles, and RCA and the newest Motorola control units. Operating instructions are also presented for area hospitals and for mobile radios.

337. Uhley, Herman N. "Electrocardiographic Telemetry from Ambulances. A Practical Approach to Mobile Coronary Care Units." American Heart Journal 80 (December 1970): 838-42.

Literature

> This report, of an experience at Mount Zion Hospital and Medical Center, San Francisco, presents one approach to a segment of coronary care which attempts, by means of electrocardiogram telemetry, to utilize the merits of mobile coronary care systems without the associated overwhelming costs.

338. Virginia. Polytechnic Institute and State University. <u>Emergency Medical Services Communications.</u> Blackburg, Va.: Department of Industrial Engineering and Operation Research, 1974. 110 p. (NTIS HRP 0004514)

> Four alternative plans were prepared for the New River Valley Planning District Emergency Medical Service Communications System. One plan assumes a decision to retain present low-band radio equipment. The other three assume a decision to go to the new HHF Federal Communication Commission channels assigned for special emergency radio service. The use of the 911 or alternate emergency telephone numbers are explored. Also, this book discusses the interface of EMS communications with other safety functions.

339. Vogt, Fred B. "Communication Systems for Emergency Medical Services. Part 1: General Description." <u>Emergency Medical Services</u> 1 (November-December 1972): 18-21, 44-45.

> The fact that emergency medical services must extend beyond the walls of the hospital to render prehospital care makes coordinated communications essential. Various types of communication are discussed, including: public education, reporting, dispatch center, emergency vehicle communication, hospital-to-hospital communications, telemetry, and paging. For communications to function, a community must organize its emergency response system. Problems in organization and implementation are discussed.

340. Werner, Martin, and Wright, Peter. <u>Emergency Medical Communications, Wisconsin 1969.</u> Madison, Wis.: Department of Health and Social Services, December 1979. 78 p.

> An inventory of and future considerations for emergency medical services communications in Wisconsin are presented. Summaries of some of the more salient features of systems in New Jersey, California, Missouri, and Nebraska are included. Future considerations for Wisconsin include: district-wide central dispatch, in-transit ambulance communication, hospital radio communications, regional communication for regional medical care, and federal funding.

C. TRANSPORTATION

An EMSS must include a necessary number of ground, air, and water emergency transportation vehicles and facilities to respond adequately to the transportation needs of the system.

Literature

All vehicles and facilities must meet standards relating to location, design, performance, and equipment, such as the federal standards KKK-A-1822 for ambulances, and equipment for ambulances recommended by the American College of Surgeons.

This component also advises on the number of personnel needed in emergency vehicles and the location of vehicles to permit an accurate response time according to the area.

This section is divided into four main parts: (1) "Transportation--General"; (2) "Ambulances"; (3) "Mobile Coronary Care Units (MCCU)", and (4) "Air Transportation, Mainly Helicopters."

General

341. Brearley, Kenneth S. "Roadside Resuscitation: A Simple Kit." The Medical Journal of Australia 1 (25 February 1978): 208-9.

> A well-organized kit of basic emergency resuscitative equipment, which a physician could carry in a car trunk, is described. This kit would prove invaluable in treating and saving the lives of victims of traffic accidents, cardiac arrest, drowning and so on.

342. Chi Systems. Development and Application of a Planning Methodology to Increase the Effectiveness of the Emergency Medical Transportation System for the Southern Maine Comprehensive Health Association. Final Report. Ann Arbor, Boston, Columbus: February 1973. 132 p. (NTIS HRP-0005921)

> The purpose of this study is to develop and apply a planning methodology to increase the effectiveness of the emergency medical transportation system of the state of Maine. This objective was developed, tested, and applied to the SMCHA region. Second, the methodology has general application so that it can be applied to the other regions of the state.

343. Fahey, M. "Pre-Hospital Trauma Management." New Zealand Medical Journal 87 (January 1978): 54-58.

> Prehospital emergency care in the United Kingdom, West Germany, Denmark, the United States, Australia, and New Zealand are briefly compared.

344. Garvin, John M., and Miller, Kathryn P. "Emergency Medical Services: Teamwork to Fight Sudden Death." Virginia Medical 107 (January 1980): 47-49.

> The availability of prompt, effective prehospital care could prevent thousands of unnecessary deaths from accidents, myocardial infarction, and others, each year.

345. Gates, William H. "Prehospital Emergency Medical Care in Ohio." Ohio State Medical Journal 74 (August 1978): 495-96.

Literature

New regulations, combined with new procedures and concepts in prehospital emergency care are increasing the importance of Ohio's emergency medical system.

346. Larson, Richard C., and Franck, Evelyn A. <u>Dispatching the Units of Emergency Service Systems Using Automatic Vehicle Location: A Computer Based Markov Hyercube Model.</u> Cambridge: MIT, Laboratory of Architecture and Planning, April 1976. 49 p.

    Automatic vehicle location (AVL) systems present to the dispatcher of emergency response units (e.g., police cars, ambulances) the estimated real time locations of units within his service area. Building on a recently developed "hyercube queuing model," this paper presents a Markov process model for computerizing the operating characteristics of the radio-dispatcher fleet operating under a policy that dispatches the closest available unit to each call for service. The model accommodates a realistic description of the service area and rather general spatial deployment policies for units.

347. McManus, William F., et al. "Prehospital Advanced Emergency Care: A Potential Pitfall." <u>Journal of Trauma</u> 18 (May 1978): 305-7.

    Skillful and effective prehospital care may alter a patient's symptoms and vital signs. Prior to such effective care, emergency room physicians were used to certain constellations of findings which reliably indicated the severity of illness or injury. If the physician is not aware of the prehospital changes which can occur, the patient may be jeopardized.

348. Mayer, Jonathan D. "Emergency Medical Service: Delays Response Time and Survival." <u>Medical Care</u> 17 (August 1979): 818-27.

    The need to minimize ambulance response time is a primary concern in the planning of emergency medical services. Patient delay in seeking medical attention and delay in ambulance dispatching are considered. The interaction of these types of delays and their impact on patient survival is studied.

349. _____. "Seattle's Paramedic Program: Geographical Distribution, Response Time, and Mortality." <u>Social Science and Medicine</u> 13D (March 1979): 45-51.

    Minimizing time to definitive care in critical emergencies is a stated goal of most emergency medical services systems. But do survival rates from emergencies vary geographically? This paper examines Seattle's Medic 1 program and its tiered response-system within this perspective.

350. Mid-Coast Comprehensive Health Planning Association. <u>Central California M.A.S.T. Program--Military Assistance to Safety and Traffic.</u> Salinas, Calif.: MAST Coordinating Committee, 1972. 88 p. (NTIS HRO-00000178)

Literature

The Mid-Coast Comprehensive Health Planning Association developed the proposal for the California Military Assistance to Safety and Traffic Coordinating Committee (MAST) to analyze the possibility of creating a more complete Emergency Medical Services System. The consultants studied the resident population in the emergency medical service area; identified the nonresident population; assessed the military and civilian resources for emergency medical service, including land and air ambulances, hospitals, communication and training facilities.

351. Mid-South Center Council for Comprehensive Health Planning. DeSoto County Emergency Medical Service Transportation Plan. Memphis, Tenn.: February 1974. 31 p. (NTIS HRO-0003753)

Conditions and projections with regard to population, traffic volume, and accidental deaths and injuries in DeSoto County, Mississippi, are described. Tables are used to display data documenting a projected increase in demand for emergency medical services (EMS) in the area over the next twenty years. Demand for service, distribution of that demand, and emergency call demand centers are discussed as components of the EMS transportation plan. Estimated capital requirements and annual operating costs for the transportation system (contract with commercial ambulance company and county-operated ambulance service) are summarized. Maps depict the emergency ambulance response times for different ambulance base location configurations. Recommendations include restricting the use of emergency ambulance vehicles for trauma or sudden illness patients through use of invalid vehicles for transporting persons who are nonambulatory but do not require medical treatment while in transit.

352. Monroe, Charles B. "A Simulation Model for Planning Emergency Response Systems." Social Science and Medicine 14D (March 1980): 71-77.

Madison, Wisconsin's, public emergency ambulance service is evaluated by means of a simulation model of emergency response system. The validity of the model, which can reproduce the events in an actual emergency response situation, is tested against a sample of emergency calls from Madison's actual system.

353. Nadler, Arnold David. "Planning the Efficient Delivery of Pre-Hospital Emergency Medical Services: A Systems Analysis." Ph.D. dissertation, Hunter College, New York, 1974. 315 p.

Models are developed for assessing policy alternatives for delivering prehospital emergency medical services, with emphasis on organizational variables for increasing system capacity efficiently in regard to rapidity of response and capability for providing on-scene and in-transit patient care. Data collected from Yale-New Haven Hospital and during visits to several ambulance systems are used to establish demand patterns for ambulance services. Among the cost

Literature

models included are systems using helicopter ambulances. Other approaches for providing improved emergency ambulance services economically are considered in examinations of variable system capacity as a function of time of day, service district population, volunteer service in rural areas, and interaction with police patrol activities.

354. National Emergency Medical Services Information Clearinghouse. <u>Emergency Medical Services: Transportation Guidelines</u>. Philadelphia: Center for the Study of Emergency Health Services, July 1976. 95 p.

    Report presents guidelines for the specific equipment and vehicles necessary to an acceptable transportation system and their operation within the total scope of the Emergency Medical Services. Provisions of the three major documents that have been generally accepted as national standards for ambulance design and equipment are outlined and the advantages and disadvantages of the various strategies for ambulance service are discussed: fire department-based; police-based; hospital-based; volunteer; commercial-private; combinations; and other unique approaches. Report also discusses merits and weaknesses of various designs for ambulances, describes mobile intensive care units, outlines use of special vehicles such as golf carts and snowmobiles, and discusses allied EMS vehicular services and strategies for ambulance location.

355. North Shore Health Planning Council. <u>Emergency Medical Transportation: A Regional System</u>. Peabody, Mass.: January 1975. 17 p. (NTIS HRP-0004016)

    Information developed in meetings held to examine emergency medical services transportation in Lynn, Peabody, Saugus, Swampscott, and Lynnfield, Massachusetts, is summarized. A regional plan which combines the emergency ambulances of these neighboring communities is shown to offer a higher level of community emergency medical care for fewer dollars than any plan requiring communities to act separately. The meeting participants--representatives of the medical community and of public safety agencies in the five towns--discussed the following issues: public perception of EMS transportation; ways in which EMS transportation could be improved; and effects of the 1973 Ambulance Law of Massachusetts. The proposed regional plan would replace six potentially obsolete vehicles with four fully staffed ambulances owned or contracted for by an independent, nonprofit EMS authority. The role of private ambulance companies and of police and fire services in the plan is outlined.

356. Sandler, R. <u>EMS Transportation Overview: Initial Results</u>. Ann Arbor, Mich.: CSF, 1974. 10 p.

    This document was prepared to analyze the requests for non-routine EMS services, and to identify possible improvement areas. Findings show that the average numbers of urgent requests per day is not substantial.

Literature

357. Silverston, Paul P. "Roadside Care and Rescue American Style." Injury 11 (August 1979): 96-98.

    This paper discusses emergency medical services system development and paramedical training in the United States.

358. _____. "Roadside Medical Care in Cambridgeshire." Injury 11 (November 1979): 90-95.

    The Mid-Anglia General Practitioner Accident Service (MAGPAS), established in 1972 to provide medical care at accident sites before the arrival of the ambulance and to assist ambulance crews with the severely injured, is discussed.

359. Williams, Phyllis M., and Shavlik, Gerald. "Geographic Patterns and Demographic Correlates of Paramedic Runs in San Bernardino, 1977." Social Science and Medicine 13D (December 1979): 273-79.

    The geographic pattern of demand for paramedic services in San Bernardino is mapped. Information was obtained about age, sex, and reason for service.

Ambulances

360. Achabal, Dale D., and Schoeman, Milton E.F. "An Examination of Alternative Emergency Ambulance Systems: Contribution from an Economic Geography Perspective." Social Science and Medicine 13D (June 1979): 81-86.

    The structure of the ambulance system operating within the emergency medical systems suprasystem is an important factor in deciding the quality and level of emergency patient care. A competitive environment has a strong influence over urban ambulance location patterns. The major choice to be made is between independent operator of emergency services or a municipally operated and/or controlled EMS system. The effect of competitive and socially optimal location patterns on patient survival and resource utilization is studied.

361. American College of Surgeons. Model Ordinance Regulating Ambulance Service. Chicago: August 1966. 24 p.

    This model ordinance for ambulance service was developed in a joint action program of the American College of Surgeons, American Association for the Surgery of Trauma, and the National Safety Council. The ordinance was intended to serve as a guide to improving ambulance services and to promote standardization of those services throughout the United States.

362. American College of Surgeons. Committee on Trauma. "Essential Equipment for Ambulances." Bulletin ACS 62 (September 1977): 7-12.

    The equipment described is considered by the Committee on Trauma to be that which is essential if the emergency medical technician is to provide adequate care for the critically ill and injured at the emergency site and during transport to medical facilities.

Literature

363. Bell, Colling E., and Allen, David. "Optimal Planning of an Emergency Ambulance Service." Socio-Economic Planning Sciences 3 (August 1969): 95-101.

    Queuing theory models are developed for determining the number of ambulances needed to serve a region. The criterion used is to provide immediate service to 95 percent or 99 percent of calls for emergency transportation. The area of the models have available only one or two units.

364. Benson, Don M., and Weigel, J.A. "Advanced Life-Support by Volunteer Fire Department Ambulance Personnel." JACEP 4 (March-April 1975): 119-22.

    A total of 95 percent of the personnel delivering emergency ambulance service in many areas of the United States are volunteers. In order to find out if such personnel can provide effective advanced life-support, the Western Pennsylvania Regional Medical Program conducted a project that trained fifteen volunteer ambulance personnel in these techniques.

365. Blum, Marc S., et al. Ambulance Placement Strategies for Emergency Medical Systems. Atlanta: Georgia Institute of Technology, January 1974. 133 p.

    This is a guide for determining ambulance locations. The user must supply such data as population by census tract, target response time by area, and mean velocity of ambulances by area. By estimation and approximation techniques, the user is taken step by step through a series of calculations to determine ambulance locations.

366. Boldt, Ronald, et al. Analysis of Ambulance Service Needs in Yuba-Sutter Counties. Chico: Superior California Comprehensive Planning Association, December 1973. 21 p. (NTIS HRP-000 4318)

    The economic feasibility of adding a third ambulance service in Sutter and Yuba Counties, as well as the impact such an addition would have on the quality of emergency medical care in those counties is considered. Existing emergency care resources in the area are evaluated, including an inventory of ambulances and equipment.

367. Boyd, David R., et al. "An Ambulance Strategy for Illinois." Illinois Medical Journal 144 (November 1973): 487-92.

    In order to make Illinois system a total emergency medical services system, an ambulance strategy was developed. This strategy has the following points: (1) build on existing medical resources; (2) consider the population density in need of ambulance services; (3) integrate highways, roads and access points for ambulance service response; and (4) account for all highway-related accidents and death.

Literature

368. Burt, John M. All Shortest Distances in Large Serial Networks. EMS Working Paper, no. 7. Los Angeles: University of California, Graduate School of Business Administration, EMS Project, April 1971. 21 p.

   This paper deals with the problem of finding the shortest distance between all pairs of nodes in a graph. The graph can be either directed or undirected. A serial cascade procedure is presented which has certain computational improvements over other shortest distance algorithms.

369. Chaiken, Jan M. Allocation of Emergency Units: Response Areas. New York: Rand Institute, December 1971. 9 p. (NTIS AD-742 396)

   The author presents an alternative to dispatching emergency vehicles by dispatching the unit based in closest proximity to the incident.

370. Chaiken, Jan M., and Gladstone, Robert J. Some Trends in the Delivery of Ambulance Services. Santa Monica, Calif.: Rand Corp., July 1974. 38 p. (R-1551-RWJF)

   Data obtained from 179 grant applications to the Robert Wood Johnson Foundation by emergency medical service agencies was compiled into a composite description of their mobile response systems in 1973 and their plans for future operations.

371. Chaiken, Jan M., and Larson, Richard C. Methods for Allocating Urban Emergency Units: A Survey. New York: Rand Institute, October 1971, 48 p. (NTIS AD-737 677)

   This work discusses the use of operations research techniques to the problem of allocating urban emergency units.

372. Cooper, Carole, et al. Description and Analysis of Eighteen Proven Emergency Ambulance Service Systems. 2 vols. Washington, D.C., DOT, 1968. (NTIS PB-179 651/652)

   This is a study to identify a range of nationwide working solutions to the emergency medical services problem, and to investigate how several communities developed their approaches to provide adequate EMS.

373. Crampton, Richard S., et al. "Amelioration of Prehospital and Ambulance Death Rates from Coronary Artery Disease by Prehospital Emergency Cardiac Care." JACEP 4 (January-February 1975): 19-23.

   This article relates a three-year period experience of community-wide prehospital cardiopulmonary resuscitation (CPR) and emergency cardiac care (ECC). It was found that hospital mortality fell to 8.8 percent and prehospital, ambulance, and community coronary death rates also declined.

374. Deems, John Michael. "Prediction of Calls for Emergency Ambulance Service." Master's thesis, Georgia Institute of Technology, Atlanta, August, 1973. 91 p.

Literature

>This research investigates the possibility of using linear regression models to predict demand for ambulance service from socioeconomic census tract data.

375. Doeksen, Gerald A., et al. Economics of Rural Ambulance in the Great Plains: A Feasibility Analysis for Local Decision-Makers. Agricultural Economic Report, no. 308. Washington, D.C.: U.S. Department of Agriculture, Economic Research Service, November 1975. 28 p.

   >The study area for this report consisted of eight counties in northwest Oklahoma, the socioeconomic data being applied to Alfalfa County specifically. A procedure to estimate receipts for Emergency Medical Service was designed from the supplied data. Expenses were based on a consideration of each major component comprising an EMS system.

376. Dunlap and Associates. Economics of Highway Emergency Ambulance Service: Final Report. 2 vols. Darien, Conn.: July 1968. (NTIS PB-178 837/838)

   >The objectives of this project are to provide a brief but accurate description of the status of ambulance services across the country, describe the operational and economic impact of recent legislation on the major types of purveyors of ambulance services, develop methods for determining the optimum density of ambulances needed to provide specified levels of service to communities or areas, develop formulae that the federal and state governments could use for computing equitable subsidies or financial support for eligible communities, and prepare guideline information that local leaders can use in identifying and evaluating alternative solutions to their specific problems in providing an emergency ambulance service.

377. Finn, Peter, and Wolff, Peter. "Learning About Emergency Vehicles." Journal of School Health 48 (December 1978): 600-602.

   >This article discusses the development of a course to prepare and teach students how to behave properly, and make the right decisions in emergency cases. The point of emphasis is how to contact and facilitate the arrival of emergency vehicles.

378. Fitzsimmons, James Albert. "Emergency Medical Systems: A Simulation Study and Computerized Method for Deployment of Ambulances." Ph.D. dissertation, University of California, Los Angeles, School of Business Administration, 1970. 207 p.

   >The author develops the mean response time model used in CALL (Computerized Ambulance Location Logic). One of the most significant contributions to this area of study is his approach to design parameters, control policies, and sensitivity analysis on mean response time.

379. _____. "Methodology for Emergency Ambulance Deployment." Management Science 19 (February 1973): 627-36.

The development of an operational deployment methodology which is based on a model of an ambulance system is described. The response time of a system ambulance for a particular call depends on the state of the system when the call is received. Often when a medical emergency occurs, the ambulance that would normally be assigned may be busy; therefore, an idle but more distant ambulance is dispatched. The model is based on response time of an actual operating system--the Computerized Ambulance Location Logic (CALL) of Los Angeles, California.

380. Gibson, Geoffrey. "Evaluative Criteria for Emergency Ambulance Systems." Social Science and Medicine 7 (1973): 425-54.

Although agencies have developed minimum standards for emergency ambulance services, systematic criteria for program evaluation are lacking. This study has examined over fifty evaluative surveys on ambulance services in the United States and abroad in an attempt to develop suitable evaluative criteria.

381. _____. "Measures of Emergency Ambulance Effectiveness: Unmet Need and Inappropriate Use." JACEP 6 (September 1977): 389-92.

Health Systems Agencies, in order to fulfill their needs assessment and facility regulation functions under the National Health Planning and Resource Development Act of 1974 (PL 93-641), process measures are needed to evaluate the overall efficiency of an emergency ambulance system. In Erie County, New York, unmet ambulance need, defined as the portion of emergency patients who clinically need ambulance transportation but do not receive it, was found to be 55 percent. Inappropriate ambulance use, the proportion of emergency patients receiving ambulance care who did not clinically need it, was found to be 30 percent.

382. Hall, William K. "The Application of Multifunction Stochastic Service Systems in Allocating Ambulances to an Urban Area." Operations Research 20 (May-June 1972): 558-70.

This article analyzes the problems of determining the allocation and distribution of ambulances within a city. A model was developed to model multifunction emergency vehicles. The model accounts for police and ambulance calls and the interaction of vehicles performing both functions. The model was used to assess distribution and assignment policies for Detroit.

383. _____. "Management Science Approaches to the Determination of Urban Ambulance Requirements." Socio-Economic Planning Sciences 5 (October 1971): 491-99.

This research paper summarizes a systematic approach to the determination of urban ambulance requirements. Quantitative measures of ambulance system performance and alternative system configurations were developed. An analy-

Literature

tical model was developed and applied to the Detroit emergency transportation system. This model was used to predict the performance of alternative system configurations under varying operating policies.

384. Hisserich, John Charles. "Public Emergency Ambulance Service: Determinants of Demand." Ph.D. dissertation, University of California, Los Angeles School of Public Health, 1971. 261 p.

    The service provided by public emergency ambulances is defined, placed into historical and contemporary perspective, and analyzed in detail for Los Angeles. A model for determining factors that may influence the demand for such service was developed. To examine possible demand relationships, a large sample of the demands on the ambulance service in Los Angeles is used as the dependent variable in a number of multiple regression analyses.

385. Holloway, Ronald M. "New York City's Experience in Improving Ambulance Service." Health Services Reports 87 (May 1972): 445-50.

    Examination of the existing ambulance system in New York revealed that many improvements could be made at no cost, such as centralized control and administration, and relocation of units to better meet call demand. EMT training was standardized and experienced nurses were utilized to evaluate incoming calls through the 911 network.

386. Javis, James P., et al. A Simple Procedure for the Allocation on Ambulances in Semi-Rural Areas. Cambridge: MIT, Innovative Resource, March 1975. 53 p. (TR-13-75)

    This joint project of MIT Innovative Resource Planning Project and the Bel-O-Mar Regional Council of Wheeling, West Virginia, developed a regional ambulance allocation plan for an area of low population density, 147 people per square mile.

387. Jelenko, Judith M., and Jelenko, Carl, III. "Change Theory in Action: The 1972 Georgia Ambulance Law." JACEP 4 (May-June 1975): 236-40.

    Change theory is applied to the goal of obtaining an ambulance law for the state of Georgia. The governor established an Emergency Medical Services Commission that led the process through legislation, regulations, systems planning, funding, and implementation. The joining of disparate individuals, groups, and organizations, assessing the problem, evaluating resources, planning the change process, creating the change, and assuring self-perpetuation of the change are examined.

388. Jensen, Ken E. "A Hospital-Based Ambulance Service." Hospitals 46 (16 March 1972): 65-69.

Literature

Jensen describes the use of a hospital-based ambulance service in Menominee, Wisconsin. It describes the planning of the service, and details the training of ambulance personnel and their integration into the hospital, agreements with law enforcement agencies, and the expenses and revenue generated by the hospital-based service. The data contained are for 1969 and 1970.

389. Kentucky. State Department of Health. Emergency Ambulance Service in Kentucky: A Report of Survey Findings and Recommendations. Frankfort, Ky.: Comprehensive Emergency Service Project, December 1970. 106 p.

   This study is the result of a survey of ambulance services in Kentucky. It reviews the origin of service, the types of vehicles and equipment used, the patterns of calls, personnel qualifications, communications, financial status, and cost of service. It also includes attitudes of providers toward the quality of service.

390. Lanoy, M., and Berge S. "Medically Equipped Emergency Ambulance Units at 'Hospital Civil de Charleroi': Four Years' Activity." Acta Anaestheslologica Belgica 3 (September 1979): 189-99.

   This article describes the emergency ambulance service provided by the Hospital of Charleroi. The ambulances are staffed on a twenty-four hour basis by five hospital physicians, who rotate responsibilities.

391. Larson, Richard C. Response of Emergency Units: The Effects of Barriers, Discrete Streets, and One-Way Streets. Rand Report, no. R-675-HUD. Final Report. New York: Rand Institute, April 1971. 31 p.

   The purpose of this program is to determine what effect barriers and one-way streets have upon response time of emergency ambulance vehicles. Mean travel distance is the measure of effectiveness.

392. Larson, Richard C., and Stevenson, Keith A. On Insensitivities in Urban Redistricting and Facility Location. Rand Report, no. R-533-NYC-HUD. Final Report. New York: Rand Institute, March 1971. 24 p.

   This paper deals with the problems of facility locations. An arbitrary urban service system is used wherein vehicles are dispatched to incidents from fixed facilities. The author demonstrates that with spatially homogeneous demands, the mean travel time resulting from a random distribution of facilities increases only 25 percent over the travel time for optimal distributed facilities.

393. Lazner, J. "Paramedical Education--The Hungarian Experience: Ambulance Attendant and Ambulance Officer Training." Medical Journal of Australia 1 (9 February 1980): 101-2.

Literature

        The article explains how the Budapest, Hungary, ambulance service was developed and how its medical practitioners, the equivalent of the American EMT, are trained.

394. Levalley, Norma. "Modified Golf Cart Goes Where Ambulance Cannot." <u>Hospital Topics</u> 46 (February 1968): 71-72.

        California State College at Los Angeles transformed a golf cart into a special-purpose ambulance to improve emergency care on campus.

395. Los Angeles. City Fire Department. <u>Emergency Rescue Ambulance Deployment Project.</u> Los Angeles: July 1973. 90 p.

        This is a simulation study of location for ambulance units in the city of Los Angeles. Based on the demography of the area, the authors apply in this model the concepts of location, queuing theory, dispatching and response times.

396. Lund, Ivar, and Skulberg, Andreas. "Experiences With a Doctor-Manned Ambulance Service in Oslo." <u>Journal of Oslo City Hospital</u> 21 (October 1971): 150-58.

        An ambulance service is an important part of modern medical service. Such a service must be organized according to the local circumstances, the available resources and the degree of achievement aimed at. The experiences with a doctor-manned ambulance service in Oslo are described. The authors believe that there are few, if any, investments in medicine, whether in personnel or direct expenses, which will guarantee such a profit in terms of lives saved and complications prevented as that spent on an efficient ambulance service.

397. McClendon, E.L., and Fikes, J.M. "Rural Ambulance Service." <u>Hospitals</u> 45 (16 April 1971): 66-68.

        The need to improve rural emergency medical services was met in a unique way in the community of Tulare, California. Identifying the weakest link in the chain of services as the ambulance service, the board of directors of the Tulare District Hospital moved the service from the fire department to the hospital. Legal, medical, political, economic, and organizational aspects are discussed.

398. Meyer, John W. "Dual Response in Rural EMS System." <u>Emergency Medical Services</u> 4 (January-February 1975): 22-24.

        This article discusses two alternatives for quality ambulance service in rural areas. The program, dual response, has proven workable in Wisconsin and can be described as an organized response that involves more vehicles and personnel than the normal response with one fully staffed vehicle.

Literature

399. Murphy, Steven P. "Organization and Management of Emergency Ambulance Care and Emergency Hospitals." International Anesthesiology Clinic 9 (1971): 189-218.

    "A synopsis is presented of the history of the development of emergency transportation and care in a large southwestern U.S. county which encompasses virtually all possible geographical areas. It also summarizes the in-hospital organization of emergency services and the inter-hospital relationships of emergency services, and gives a description of our phased transportation plan currently under development. It also summarizes our experience with helicopter ambulances and our proposed use of these vehicles for limited local disasters."

400. National Academy of Sciences-National Research Council. Division of Medical Sciences. Committee on Emergency Medical Services. Medical Requirements for Ambulance Design and Equipment. Public Health Service Publication, no. 1071-C-3. Washington, D.C.: Government Printing Office, 1970. 24 p.

    This document generally describes the ambulance design and equipment necessary for prehospital medical care. Chapters include: "The Ambulance: Security and Rescue Equipment"; "Emergency Care Equipment and Supplies"; "Communication"; and Documentation and Transportation by Air."

401. Perrine, Edward L., and Hall, David S. "Rural Ambulance Service Characteristics and Demands Without Economic Barriers." Appalachia Medicine 4 (Winter 1972): 86-93.

    This is a study of demand for ambulance services in a rural West Virginia county where service is provided by a funeral home. The study reports on the demographic and financial characteristics of users of the service and compares these variables during control periods with a period in which financial barriers to use are removed.

402. Pozen, Michael W., et al. "Cost and Utility Considerations in Implementing Ambulance Telemetry." Heart and Lung 9 (September-October 1980): 866-71.

    This paper presents a step-by-step method which emergency medical service administrators can use to assess the potential benefits of telemetry in their communities.

403. Safar, Peter, et al. "Ambulance Design and Equipment for Mobile Intensive Care." Archives of Surgery 102 (March 1971): 163-71.

    The authors, based on their fourteen years of experience with ambulance design and equipment, recommend: (1) national standards could be implemented at the local level; (2) existing assembly line vehicles could be further transformed into mobile intensive care units at relatively low cost; and (3) the equipment recommended and described has proved valuable in actual practice.

Literature

404. Savas, E.S. "Simulation and Cost-Effectiveness Analysis of New York's Emergency Ambulance Service." Management Science 15 (August 1969): B-600-627.

    A computer simulation was used to analyze possible improvements in the New York ambulance service.

405. Scanlan, Larry. "Rushing Roulette: The State of Canada's Ambulance Service." Canadian Family Physician 22 (February 1976): 61-77.

    In a Canada-wide survey, Canadian Family Physician found a startling divergence in provincial standards for ambulance crews and vehicles. While some provinces had developed a well-integrated ambulance system with central dispatching, rigorous standards for attendants and advanced paramedical training programs, in some the ambulances are run almost entirely by local morticians.

406. Schneider, Jerry B., and Symons, John G., Jr. Locating Ambulance Dispatch Centers in an Urban Region: A Computer Interactive Problem-Solving Approach. RSRI Discussion Paper Series, no. 49. Philadelphia: Regional Science Research Institute, July 1971. 40 p.

    A computerized system for solving the ambulance location problem is described. The system is called ADLOC, Ambulance Dispatch Center Location.

407. Scott, David W., et al. "Predicting the Response Time of an Urban Ambulance System." Health Services Research 13 (Winter 1978): 404-17.

    A model was developed in order to predict the response time of an urban ambulance system. The model was tested using data collected from ambulance runs in Houston, Texas. The authors report a close agreement between model predicted and real ambulance response time.

408. Siler, Kenneth F. "Predicting Demand for Publicly Dispatched Ambulances in a Metropolitan Area." Health Services Research 10 (1975): 254-63.

    A model is described for predicting ambulance demand, based on data from Los Angeles County ambulance system. An estimated 2.4 million visits were made between June 1973 and June 1974 to approximately 190 emergency facilities in Los Angeles County.

409. Smalley, Harold E. Ambulance Placement Strategies for Emergency Medical Systems. Atlanta: Georgia Institute of Technology, Health Research Systems Center, January 1974. 144 p. (NTIS PB-242 084)

    The report is a programmed planning guide for emergency medical planners in determining ambulance placement strategies. It provides a comprehensive plan of technical systems capabilities for identifying problems associated with the provision of emergency medical services in the metropolitan Atlanta area. It discusses the requirement for number, types, and

Literature

geographical positioning of emergency vehicles; a recommendation of an organization for coordination; operation, and control of the EMS system component; a communication subsystem design; a comprehensive set of procedures for performing the dispatch and control function; recommendation for training EMS personnel; a scheme for evaluation; EMS system performance; and recommendation for financing of the EMS system.

410. Stevenson, Keith Allister. Operational Aspects of Emergency Ambulance Service. Cambridge: MIT, Operations Research Center, May 1971. 162 p. (TR-No. 61)

   A primary and secondary ambulance model is developed. Ambulance service is provided from a single source, primary model, or from a combination of two sources, secondary model. In the secondary model, a primary source dispatches ambulances as long as they are available. Costs for this service is a linear function of the number of ambulances used. When the primary source is exhausted, a secondary source can be called upon at fixed cost per call.

411. Swoveland, C.D., et al. "Ambulance Location: A Probabilistic Enumeration Approach." Management Science 20 (December 1973): 686-98.

   A simulation technique is developed for determining the optimal location of ambulances. The approach consists of dividing the geographic area into a series of zones. Each zone is approximated by a central point or node. Regions are formed by grouping nodes. The objective is to locate one ambulance in each region. The procedure determines at which node within a region the ambulance should be located so that the total average response time is minimized.

412. Texas. Municipal League. Ambulance Service in Texas. Austin: December 1972. 126 p.

   This a set of guidelines for municipal officers in decision making about alternative approaches to provide adequate ambulance services in Texas.

413. Toregas, Constantine, and ReVelle, Charles. "Optimal Location Under Time or Distance Constraints." Papers of the Regional Science Association 28 (1972): 133-43.

   A justification for using minimum time as a surrogate measure for social utility in urban location problems is presented. A thesis is presented for a constraint on the maximum time which separates a user from a facility and an optimization problem is formulated to minimize the number of facilities subject to this constraint.

414. Torrey, E. Fuller. "Emergency Psychiatric Ambulance Services in The USSR." American Journal of Psychiatry 128 (August 1971): 153-57.

Literature

In 1965, psychiatrists in the Soviet Union began an experiment in emergency psychiatric ambulance services. This system has the following advantages: immediate treatment is provided; physicians rather than police bring patients to the hospital; information can be gathered from witnesses at the crisis scene; and feldshers (medical workers) assist psychiatrists. The author raises several questions about the provision of emergency psychiatric services in the United States and concludes that we have much to learn from psychiatrists abroad.

415. U.S. Department of Transportation. National Highway Traffic Safety. Committee on Ambulance Design Criteria. Ambulance Design Criteria. Washington, D.C.: Government Printing Office, 1973. 42 p.

These criteria predate and are in general accord with federal specifications KKK-A-1822. This report is divided into two sections. Part 1 provides historical and technical background and describes the resulting need for ambulance design and performance standards. Part 2 contains specific design criteria in a system description format.

416. U.S. General Services Administration. Federal Supply Service. General Services Administration. Ambulance: Emergency Medical Care Vehicle. Federal Specifications KKK-A-1822. Washington, D.C.: January 1974. 39 p.

All institutions that intend to use federally originated monies to obtain ambulances have to comply with these specifications.

417. Volz, Richard A. "Optimun Ambulance Location in Semi-Rural Areas." Transportation Science 5 (May 1971): 193-203.

This article describes a study conducted in Washtenaw County, Michigan. The objectives of the study were to produce an ambulance location model which would minimize mean response time to an emergency call and maximize use of ambulance service.

418. Waller, Julian A., and Jacobs, Lee. Ambulance Service in Vermont. Burlington, Vt.: State Department of Health, 1970. 40 p.

This publication is the result of the 1970 survey of ambulance services.

419. West, Irvan M., et al. "Emergency Transportation: A Survey of California Ambulance Operations." California Medicine 116 (February 1972): 35-43.

The most urgent recommendation expressed by physicians, Red Cross officials, ambulance operators, and others polled in this survey was to make much more emergency medical care training available to ambulance personnel. Very few sick and injured receive first aid before an ambulance arrives. Therefore, there is also an urgent need to train and motivate

Literature

the public to provide first aid at the scene of the emergency. Urban ambulances usually respond within ten minutes, but often rural ambulances take more than thirty minutes to reach an emergency. It is during this interim that lives which could be saved by prompt first aid are lost. Little use has been made of aircraft as emergency ambulances; in 1968, only one emergency trip in fifteen hundred was made by helicopter. Also, California has fewer ambulances which make fewer emergency trips on a population basis than the country at large.

Mobile Coronary Care Units (MCCU)

420. Cameron, Margaret, et al. "Follow-Up of Emergency Ambulance Calls in Nottingham: Implications for Coronary Ambulance Service." British Medical Journal (15 February 1975): 384-86.

> Information about patients in ambulance service records has been linked to that in the patients' hospital records in an attempt to make the most efficient use of a special ambulance service for patients suspected of having heart attacks. During one week, 248 emergency (999) calls for an ambulance were made by the public in the city of Nottingham. The quality of information given to the ambulance center was poor, and all four patients eventually found to have had a myocardial infarction were described as having collapsed. A further study of patients who were also described as having collapsed has led to a system which allows an ambulance controller to send a coronary ambulance only in answer to those emergency calls where there is a reasonable possibility that the patient has had a heart attack.

421. Crampton, Richard. "Prehospital Emergency Cardiac Care in Virginia: Five Years of Progress." Virginia Medical 107 (April 1980): 312-14.

> The development of the Commonwealth of Virginia five years' prehospital emergency cardiac care system, including standards of performance and procedures for certifying and recertifying emergency medical technicians, are described.

422. Czachowski, Ralph E., et al. "The Effectiveness of Mobile Coronary Care in a Nonurban Area." JACEP 5 (July 1976): 501-4.

> A study focusing on the effectiveness of a mobile coronary care unit serving a primarily semirural area of Pennsylvania was carried out over an eight-month period. During that time the unit served 225 suspected cardiac patients. A total of 29 persons died either before reaching the hospital or in the emergency department; 105 persons were placed in the intensive coronary care unit; and 42 were discharged home. Prehospital treatment definitely saved 8 lives, 3 for the long-term and 5 short-term.

Literature

423. Dyer, N.H. <u>Guidelines for Mobile Intensive Care Paramedics.</u> Charleston, W. Va.: State Department of Health, 1973. 35 p.

    General regulations concerning procedures and requirements for becoming a Mobile Intensive Care Paramedic and formulated by the West Virginia State Department of Health. Following completion of the EMT training, the paramedic trainee must undergo clinical training in either the intensive care unit, the coronary care unit, or the emergency department.

424. Frank, H.D., et al. "Ambulance with Intensive Care Facilities for the Transport of Infants at Risk." <u>Journal of Perinatal Medicine</u> 2 (1973): 125-32.

    Newborns with ongoing disturbances in vital functions following primary resuscitation in the delivery room often must be transferred over long distances to pediatric or neonatal intensive care units. Continuation of therapy, monitoring, and nursing care once initiated may prove to be quite difficult and even dangerous for both patient and accompanying medical personnel during a hasty trip with an inadequately secured narrow transport incubator. Drawing on prior experience gained both in Germany and other countries, the physicians and technicians of the Children's Clinic of the Free University of Berlin in West Berlin developed an emergency transport service for newborns that meets the prerequisites of perinatal emergencies with regard to personnel staffing, equipment outfitting, and purposeful organization.

425. Lewis, Richard P., et al. "The Columbus Emergency Medical Service System." <u>Ohio State Medical Journal</u> 75 (June 1979): 391-94.

    This is a description of the Columbus, Ohio, Fire Department Emergency Medical Services. This system is considered one of the most sophisticated and cost-effective operation in the United States.

426. Luger, G.W., and Kolsters, W. "Preliminary Experience with a Mobile Coronary Care Unit, Cardulance." <u>Folia Medica Neerlandica</u> 14 (1971): 187-95.

    The first fifteen weeks of operation are described for a mobile coronary care unit, Cardulance, that was put into service by two hospitals in the Netherlands city of Utrech during January 1971. The effectiveness of the MCCU in meeting patient needs is discussed, and the unit's layout and method of operation are detailed. It is noted that an adequately equipped mobile coronary care unit such as the Cardulance requires a highly qualified crew with considerable experience in coronary care.

427. MacMahon, A.G. "Four Years' Experience with South Africa's First Mobile Accident Unit." <u>South African Medical Journal</u> 53 (4 March 1978): 333-37.

The facts and figures relating to the four years' experience
are divided into three categories: incidents, patients and
injuries, and treatment. The wider implications for using
such a unit are also considered.

428. Marcus, Howard, and Crampton, Richard S. "Rural Mobile Coronary
Care." *Virginia Medical Monthly* 191 (February 1974): 126-28.

A rural mobile coronary care unit was established in the
town of Haysi in the coal-mining region of the Appalachian
Mountains, southwest Virginia. This article describes a
family physician's system for prehospital emergency cardiac
care in a rural community without a hospital. The need for
public education is emphasized.

429. Murtomaa, Markku, and Korttila, K. "Experience of Cardiopulmonary
Resuscitation Outside Hospital by a Mobile Intensive Care Unit."
Resuscitation 3, no. 57 (1974): 211-14.

The mobile intensive care unit was called to 770 patients
in Helsinki, of whom 85 were clinically dead. Of the 770,
cardiopulmonary resuscitation was attempted in 77 cases, but
only 4 survived long-term, compared with 12 patients of the
175 previously treated in the hospital emergency department,
but not by the MICU.

430. Nussenfeld, Sidney, et al. "Mobile Coronary Care Units: A Preliminary Critique." *Journal of the Florida Medical Association* 57 (November 1970): 17-21.

Mobile coronary care unit models existing in 1970 are described briefly and the use and effectiveness of mobile units
is assessed subjectively. The models are as follows: (1)
the Belfast, Ireland, model, using an ambulance staffed by
a physician, nurse, and possibly a medical student and
equipped to defibrillate and catheterize; (2) the Moscow,
USSR, model, involving ambulances staffed by physicians
and nurses and equipped to handle cardiac cases of different levels of severity; (3) the St. Vincent's Hospital model
(New York City), using an ambulance staffed by a team of
seven and equipped to set up a coronary care unit at the
location where the patient is found; and (4) the Miami, Florida, models, which respond to all human injury or illness
alarms but do not generally transport patients to hospitals.

431. Pantridge, J. Frank, and Adgey, A.A. Jennifer. "Prehospital Coronary Care: The Mobile Coronary Care Unit." *American Journal of Cardiology* 24 (November 1969): 666-72.

The majority of deaths from myocardial infarction occur soon
after the onset of symptoms and before the victims reach
hospital coronary care units. The mobile scheme described
allows intensive care to commence in the patient's own home
or at the site of infarction and thus reduces considerably
the interval between the onset of symptoms and the initiation

Literature

of intensive care. The prevention of fatal dysrhythmias by early prehospital care should have a significant effect on the early high mortality rates. Since the correction of ventricular fibrillation outside the hospital is a practical proposition, a further impact on the early high mortality will result when mobile units are supported by first aid training programs in methods of resuscitation.

432. Pyo, Yoon H., and Watts, Richard W. "Mobile Coronary Care Unit: An Evaluation for its Need." Annals of Internal Medicine 73 (July 1970): 61-66.

   An evaluation is described of patterns of care for acute myocardial infarction patients at a west-side hospital in Cleveland, Ohio, preliminary to a decision regarding establishment of a new MCCU. The greatest delay in care of the acute myocardial infarcted patient was found to result from the patient's unwillingness to call for help. Study findings were assessed to indicate that the existing transportation system was adequate.

433. Sherman, Mark A. "An Evaluation of the Effectiveness of Mobile Intensive Care Units in Reducing Deaths to Myocardial Infarction." Master's thesis, Northwestern University, Evanston, Illinois, June 1977. 299 p.

   Four communities which have introduced mobile intensive care units (MICUs) during the past five years were studied. The independent variable was the presence or absence of a community-wide mobile intensive care system. The dependent variable was the mortality rate for acute myocardial infarction. The research design used was a multiple interrupted time series quasiexperiment. Data was obtained from hospital medical records. Analysis showed a statistically significant decrease in mortality in two of the study communities. Plausible rival hypothesis were examined to see if other factors than the introduction of the MICUs could have led to the changes observed.

434. _____. "Mobile Intensive Care Units: An Evaluation of Effectiveness." JAMA 241 (4 May 1979): 1897-1901.

   This paper presents a retrospective evaluation of the impact of the implementation of mobile intensive care units in four suburban communities on patient outcome. Two communities exhibited a statistically significant decline in mortality rates after inception of service; the reduction of the third community was not significant. In the fourth community, the mortality rate increased.

435. Thompson, R.G., et al. "Ambulance Life Support and Outcome of Cardiovascular Emergencies." Heart and Lung 8 (May-June 1979): 486-94.

This paper analyzes the Houston ambulance life-support system and its effectiveness in reducing cardiovascular deaths. Unexpected findings let the authors to believe the ambulance life-support system may not be beneficial to some patients.

Air Transportation

436. Air Medical Evacuation System (AMES) Demonstration Project. 3 vols. Final Report. Tempe: Arizona State University, College of Engineering and Sciences, May 1970. (NTIS PB-193 724/725)

    One approach to the post-crash problem of reducing the numbers of deaths and permanent injuries is to provide the earliest possible first aid, rescue, emergency transportation, and competent medical care for persons involved in motor vehicle accidents. If such measures are taken, the resulting mortality and morbidity rates can be reduced. This is particularly appropriate for remote and rural areas, where death follows injury with the greatest frequency. AMES, which incorporates the helicopter, well-trained paramedical personnel, and well-designed communications system, was developed and tested in 1969 by the Arizona State University under a U.S. DOT demonstration project contract.

437. Burghart, Hans. "The Use of Helicopters as Mobile Intensive Units in Disaster Control and Rescue Service in the Federal Republic." Resuscitation 3 (1974): 143-45.

    Since the establishment of a rescue helicopter service in the Federal German Republic, between November 1970 and May 31, 1974, about ten thousand missions were flown. Seventy-five hundred patients received first aid at the scene of the accident; twenty-five hundred cases, of which seven hundred were potential fatalities, were transported by the helicopter to the hospital.

438. Cooper, Mary Ann, et al. "A Hospital-Based Helicopter Service: Will it Fly?" Annals of Emergency Medicine 9 (September 1980): 451-55.

    A successful experience of one hospital-based helicopter service is presented. Included are guidelines for financial feasibility study and implementation of a helicopter transport system.

439. Cowley, R. Adams, et al. "An Economical and Proven Helicopter Program for Transporting the Critically Ill and Injured Patient in Maryland." Journal of Trauma 13 (December 1973): 1029-38.

    This article describes a joint program between the Maryland State Police and the University of Maryland to supply helicopter transport of emergencies to the University of Maryland Center for the Study of Trauma. The program, put into operation in 1969, is called the Maryland Air Med-Evac Helicopter System. Four helicopter bases are used, each helicopter serving a geographic area. The units are used for:

Literature

transportation of emergency patients from the scene of the incident, interhospital transfer, transportation of medical personnel to the emergency scene or to other hospitals, and transport of equipment, supplies, blood, and organs for transplant.

440. Flexer, Morton. "The Helicopter Ambulance: Essential Medical Service." Hospital Progress 61 (May 1980): 66-71.

    The helicopter is the air ambulance of choice because it is maneuverable; requires short take-off and landing space; and it is able to hover over inaccessible sites and to land virtually anywhere. It is also faster than conventional ambulances.

441. Helicopter Ambulance Service to Emergencies (HASTE). Minneapolis, Minn.: Department of Health, March 1971. 150 p. (NTIS PB-200 308)

    The main conclusions are: (1) helicopter ambulance service in a large metropolitan area such as Minneapolis-Saint Paul, and suburbs is not feasible because of the limited operational area; (2) helicopter ambulance service would be reasonable in the outlying areas of the state.

442. Jessen, K., and Hagelsten, J.O. "S-61 Helicopter as Mobile Intensive Care Unit." Aerospace Medicine 45 (1974): 1071-74.

    Since the Sikorsky S-61 Helicopter was introduced in the Royal Danish Air Force in 1966, more than eighteen hundred missions have been carried out. Now 85 percent of the missions are for civilian purposes and the Search and Rescue Service has to be considered a king of Mobile Intensive Care Unit Service. The cabin in the S-61 Helicopter gives ample space for observation and treatment of the patient. The results of 190 missions during the last twenty-four months are evaluated. Patients suffering from heart-lung, abdominal, or intracranial diseases, and from burns or poisoning represent about 70 percent of these missions. Since vital functions cannot be monitored in the usual way in a helicopter, it was necessary to develop a dependable and safe method for continuous observation of the heart function via an ECG on an oscilloscope. The described system is relatively simple and makes continuous ECG casette recordings during flight for telemetry, later study, and interpretation possible.

443. Jordan, Robert F., Jr., et al. Planning a Helicopter Transportation System to Augment Emergency and Regional Medical Programs in a Test Region of West Virginia. Morgantown: West Virginia University, Department of Civil Engineering, 1970. 109 p. (PB 195-801)

    This is a simulation study of the potential costs and benefits of a helicopter EMS evacuation system in the rural areas around Huntington, West Virginia. Several different modes of helicopter and ground ambulance systems were simulated and compared with respect to response time, transfer time, cost, and ability to respond. The best system consists of utilizing the helicopter primarily for such functions as police patrol, medical team transfer, or reserve military training, and diverting it to emergency missions when required.

444. Josey, James Larry. "Helicopter Utilization Index for the Transport of Medical Emergencies of Highway Accidents." Ph.D. dissertation, State Colleges, Mississippi, Mississippi State University, Department of Civil Engineering, August 1970. 100 p.

    This study presents a method by which a state or political subdivision can decide whether an air ambulance would be a useful addition to an existing EMS system. A model was developed to predict the number of calls in an area per unit of time and the percentage of time-critical calls was found.

445. Mackenzie, Colin F., et al. "Two-Year Mortality in 760 Patients Transported by Helicopter Direct from the Road Accident Scene." American Surgeon 45 (February 1979): 101-8.

    This article analyzes the usage of a helicopter transport service to reduce mortality at the Maryland Institute for Emergency Medical Services.

446. Melenson, Richard S. Military Assistance to Safety and Traffic (MAST) Procedural Guide. Augusta: Southeast Georgia Hospital Association, Civilian MAST Coordinating Committee, 1975. 30 p.

    A procedural guide is presented for users of the MAST patient evacuation services in coastal Georgia and South Carolina. Through this program, the Department of the Army, Fort Stewart, Georgia, has flown over one-hundred emergency missions in support of the emergency medical services systems in the area. The MAST concept and mission are described, and procedures set forth in detail for interhospital and accident scene transfer.

447. Moylan, Joseph A. "Civilian Aeromedical Transportation: Medical Indications and Contraindications." Journal of the Kansas Medical Society 75 (December 1974): 345-48.

    With proper planning, careful selection, and suitable preparation of the patient, critically ill and injured individuals can be safely transported by air both from the initial site of the injury to the primary treatment facility, and later to a medical center with specialized capabilities for treating major trauma or complicated medical illnesses. Increasing use of aeromedical transportation will improve the delivery of coordinated medical care to critically ill and injured patients, and permit maximum utilization of specialized medical units.

448. Neumann, Edward S., et al. "Helicopter Emergency Medical Care Delivery Systems." Transportation Engineering Journal 99 (November 1973): 827-43.

Literature

This is a simulation study of the potential applicability of helicopter units in the EMS transportation system of the areas around Huntington, West Virginia.

449. Oxer, H.F. "Aeromedical Evacuation of the Seriously Ill." <u>British Medical Journal</u> 3 (1975): 692-94.

Almost any patient may be carried by air, but air transportation introduces some special problems owing to the effects of altitude, noise, turbulence, and the special environment. Because of these factors, it is important to know, when considering a patient's suitability for air transport, the type of aircraft to be used, the flight profile--its duration and expected cabin altitudes--and the facilities available on board. It is essential to carry all equipment (as simple and as portable as possible),drugs and diets that may be needed, and to be sure that all the skills and nursing help needed to deal with any possible problems are available.

450. Parker, Frank E. <u>Helicopters in Emergency Medical Services: NHTSA Experience to Date.</u> Washington, D.C.: U.S. DOT, National Highway Traffic Safety Administration, December 1972. 27 p. (DOT HS 820-231)

This paper has the purpose of documenting the efforts by the National Highway Traffic Safety Administration to study the role of the helicopter in emergency medical services. A five-year period, 1968 to 1972, is documented by excerpts from final contracts' reports. The author gives an overview of the program and comments on each particular case.

451. Peden, Guy T., et al. <u>Extension of Project CARE-SOM Coordinated Accident Rescue Endeavor, State of Mississippi.</u> State College: Mississippi State University, College of Business and Industry, Division of Research, June 1971. 215 p.

The major objective of this project was to develop a coordinated statewide helicopter-ground ambulance service. The helicopter was to be used for police traffic services. The helicopter was found to have better response time to traffic accidents, and worse time for interhospital transfers than ground ambulances.

452. Perry, I.C. "The Helicopter as a Civilian Emergency Vehicle." <u>Injury</u> 3 (April 1972): 254-56.

Helicopters have not been much used in Britain for medical purposes. Replies to questions sent to 128 hospitals and to all the police forces suggest that the medical profession is inadequately aware of the uses and limitations of helicopters. Better understanding of these matters may lead to increasing calls for helicopters in Britain; if so, the proper response to a responsible call for increased facilities would be to increase the facilities and not to stifle the calls.

Literature

453. Pettet, Gary, et al. "An Analysis of Air Transport Results in the Sick Newborn Infant: Part 1. The Transport Team." Pediatrics 55 (June 1975): 774-82.

> Regionalization of neonatal intensive care has created the need of air transport of the critically ill infant in sparsely populated areas. All newborn air transports to four Denver-area newborn intensive care units over a fourteen-month period were reviewed. An emergency-care nurse and a neonatal intensive-care nurse provided the basic transport team with physician assistance in selected cases. Infants were evaluated and stabilized at the referring hospital before moving the infant. The transports were analyzed for the type of aircraft utilized, reason for referral, and mortality. The results indicate that prior planning will permit the use of the most appropriate aircraft and transport team. When using well-trained transport personnel, the presence of a physician may be limited to specific situations without adversely affecting overall neonatal mortality.

454. Proctor, Herbert J., and Acai, Stephen A., Jr. "Assets and Liabilities of Helicopter Evacuation in Support of Emergency Medical Services." JACEP 4 (November-December 1975): 543-47.

> This article reviews the North Carolina MAST program and evaluates the helicopter's part in altering patient morbidity and mortality. One-year experience results showed that overall morbidity was reduced in 38 percent of cases evacuated. Most of the cases were cardiac problems. Mortality did not seem to be affected by using a helicopter. The shortened transfer time appeared to be more of a factor in survival than inflight care.

455. Samuels, Allen. Military Assistance to Safety and Traffic (MAST) Operations Manual. Salinas, Calif.: Mid-Coast Comprehensive Health Planning Association, MAST Coordinating Committee, 1975. 22 p.

> The utilization of military medical evacuation resources to supplement the existing EMS system and the search and rescue program in a fifteen-county, central California area is described. MAST program consists of provision of military helicopters equipped and manned as air ambulances in the event of emergencies. The helicopters serve within a one-hundred-nautical mile radius from Fort Ord, where the Army's 237th Medical Detachment is stationed. The manual describes all utilization procedures.

456. Shearman, David J., and Limmer, Allan N. "A Mantle of Safety: The 50th Year of the Royal Flying Doctor Service." British Medical Journal 2 (2 August 1978): 407-9.

> This is a description of fifty years' developments in Australia's "Royal Flying Doctor Service."

457. Skogman, David P. "The Role of Helicopters in Emergency Medical Care Systems." Master's thesis, Texas A & M University, College Station, 1971. 42 p.

Literature

The main purpose of this thesis is to contribute toward improved medical care. The results of helicopter performance in civilian air rescue operations are presented. Suggestions as to the future role of helicopters within the emergency care system are examined and recommendations are offered to aid in their improvement.

458. Stanford Research Institute. Evaluation of Operations and Marginal Costs of MAST Alternatives. Final Report. Menlo Park, Calif.: October 1971. 205 p. (NTIS AD-892 509L)

    This report is an evaluation of the operation and costs of the MAST program. Some of the results indicate that the more planning and preparation that was done, the more MAST was utilized. The more complex the chain of command, the less MAST was utilized. Cost seems to be low. The MAST alternatives are superior to a civilian operated system.

459. Stensrud, Richard L. "Hospital-Based Air Ambulance Service Extends Emergency Care." Hospital Progress 61 (May 1980): 72-77.

    In March 1978, St. Louis University Hospital began the first air rescue service in the area. With this service, the hospital system also became the region's first emergency medical services system center.

460. Turner, H.S., and Ellingson, H.V. "Use of the Helicopter as an Emergency Vehicle in the Civilian Environment: Results of a Survey-Questionnaire." Aerospace Medicine 41 (February 1970): 135-38.

    Eighty-four medical schools, fifty state highway patrols, and twelve private hospitals were surveyed by questionnaire to gather information regarding the present status and the anticipated need for the utilization of the helicopter in civilian medical care. There was general recognition by medical and police agencies of a need for helicopter transportation in certain situations. The actual utilization in the civilian community is, however, extremely limited and among the active programs the majority rely upon the military forces or Coast Guard for helicopters and crews.

461. Welch, Benjamin. "Some Considerations Before Using the Aerial Ambulance." JACEP 6 (April 1977): 155-57.

    The use of aerial ambulances for moving patients to hospitals requires some special clinical considerations. Various altitudes produce clinical problems. The Federal Aviation Agency has requirements for equipment. Factors to be considered in selecting the mode of transporting an emergency patient include patient's condition, weather, and landing location at destination. There are limitations as well as advantages in using aerial ambulances.

462. Wood, A. Michael. "Flying Doctor Services." Injury 10 (February 1979): 170-74.

Among the most important functions of this service in East Africa are dealing with medical emergencies at the scene of the accident, or evacuating patients to a medical center.

D. FACILITIES

An Emergency Medical Services System must provide an adequate number of easily accessible emergency medical services facilities which are collectively capable of providing service on a continuous and permanent basis. These facilities have to be nonduplicative and categorized according to their capabilities. These capabilities are required to meet certain appropriate standards relating to capacity, location, personnel and equipment. These facilities have to be coordinated with other health care facilities of the system.

In this bibliography we emphasize two main aspects of these facilities: (1) "Categorization," and (2) "Utilization."

Categorization

463. Agisim, Elliot. Emergency Care Capabilities of Wisconsin Hospitals: 1973 Categorization Study Report. Madison, Wis.: Department of Health and Social Services, 1973. 99 p.

> This study of categorization in Wisconsin was completed by the Bureau of Health Statistics, Section on Statistical Services, in response to state and area-wide EMS planning and development needs. It addresses four objectives: (1) to classify all Wisconsin hospital emergency departments using AMA guidelines; (2) to determine where specialized treatment centers exist; (3) to determine guidelines for accessibility of both specialized and general emergency services; and (4) to relate these guidelines to regional needs identified in the state plan. The study gives an overview of categorization in other states and presents in detail the structure of the planning organization in Wisconsin. Categorization is stressed more than regionalization, using the AMA guidelines as a measurement tool for improvement of facilities to meet the standards.

464. American Hospital Association. Categorization of Hospital Emergency Services: Report of a Conference. Chicago: 1973. 20 p.

> In December 1972, the American Hospital Association sponsored a conference to deliberate the pros and cons of categorizing hospital emergency services. The participants discuss the concept and philosophy of categorization as it pertains to urban and rural areas; the implications of categorization as it affects all aspects of the hospital and its patients, legal considerations, economic impact, transportation and communication; the categories themselves; and the development of a categorization program. The conclusions and recommendations of the conference participants are summarized and the various strategies for improving emergency medical services in a region are reviewed.

Literature

465. American Medical Association. Commission of Emergency Medical Services. <u>Categorization of Hospital Emergency Capabilities. Report of the Conference on the Guidelines.</u> Chicago: 1971. 30 p.

> This pamphlet contains guidelines developed at a conference convened by the AMA in February 1971. It recommends classification of hospital emergency services into four categories of capability: (1) comprehensive, (2) major, (3) general, and (4) basic. Each category is to meet specific criteria as to essential staff, equipment, blood bank, laboratory services, radiological services, operating rooms, postoperative recovery units, intensive care units, communications equipment, and helicopter landing facilities. The purpose of the guidelines is to identify the readiness of the hospital and its staff to receive and treat correctly all emergency patients.

466. American Society of Anesthesiology. "Community-Wide Emergency Medical Services. Recommendations by the Committee on Acute Medicine." <u>Journal of the American Medical Association</u> 204 (13 May 1968): 133-40.

> This article presents one of the first statements of criteria for categorization of hospital emergency services. Recommendations are made for total hospital facilities with the understanding that any emergency department must depend upon back-up facilities.

467. Bascomb Associates. <u>An Assessment of the Kinds of Measures (and their Availability) Required to Determine the Impact of Categorization on Hospital Finance.</u> Silver Spring, Md.: 1975. 51 p.

> The Bascomb Associates' approach for defining measures of the impact of categorization of emergency department facilities on hospital finance was to focus on data available from individual hospital department utilization rates, costs and revenue, and relate these data to patients treated in or admitted through the emergency department. Sources of data utilized to measure impact are: patient medical and billing records, hospital departmental cost and monthly utilization reports, hospital departments' monthly budget operation reports, and hospital business office reports. Any data collection for financial impact should include data over a period of three years prior to implementation of categorization and one year post-categorization.

468. _____. <u>Considerations Which are Relevant to the Methodology for Measuring the Financial Impact of Categorization.</u> Silver Spring, Md.: December 1974. Var. pag.

> This report describes a conceptual framework for selecting and evaluating hospital financial data which are relevant to measuring financial impact of categorization. Data sources for impact measurement, impact variables, charges versus costs, structural changes, and system costs are examined.

Literature

469. _____. Development and Application of a Methodology for Reviewing Areas of the County Where Categorization is Claimed to Have Taken Place. Silver Spring, Md.: November 1974. 36 p.

> This document reports on a study of published materials relating to state and regional claims for categorization. Forty-nine state and regional EMS system plans were reviewed and the data collected were subjected to two levels of evaluation. Level 1 was the extent to which an EMS system plan and categorization scheme had progressed as measured by a scale of ten criteria or major milestones for implementing a categorization scheme. Level 2 consisted of classifying each scheme in terms of a standard, using the AMA guidelines as the most widely recognized criteria for comparison.

470. Benson, Don M., and Safar, Peter. "Categorization and Regionalization of Hospital Emergency Facilities." In Public Health Aspects of Critical Care Medicine and Anesthesiology, edited by Peter Safar, pp. 138-590. Philadelphia: F.A. Davis, 1974.

> Based on a 1969 feasibility study of hospital facilities in Allegheny County (Pittsburgh, Pa.), five categories of emergency facilities are recommended: (1) comprehensive, (2) major, (3) general, (4) basic, and (5) life support station. The categories represent the views of the authors and an amalgamation of concepts presented by many others, since the study preceded the availability of the AMA guidelines. The report advocates study of all critical care areas of all hospitals, giving a total capability for vital system maintenance and definitive therapy and supports the idea that categorization of emergency services must encompass all life-threatening situations including trauma and disease.

471. Blum, Thomas H., and Walker, William. "The University Hospital in Regional Categorization." JACEP 6 (September 1977): 422-24.

> This position paper assumes the following:
>
> 1. Categorization of hospital emergency services in some form is in the best interest of the patient. Data on the effects of categorization are still soft. The hypothesis of decreased morbidity and mortality has not been proven by solid randomized studies.
>
> 2. The university medical center's role, in addition to providing definitive care, must be to evaluate critically delivery of emergency care in its community and region. If university medical centers default in this, an opportunity for a rational evolution of emergency medical systems will be lost.
>
> 3. Categorization of hospital emergency services focuses on the resources necessary to deal with approximately 5 percent of patients entering the emergency medical system.
>
> 4. Categorization of hospital emergency services, although difficult, is easier (i.e., more acceptable politically and economically than categorization or regionalization of other health care resources).

Literature

5. Categorization and regionalization of hospital emergency services are easier to implement in sparsely populated areas with a few health professionals and hospitals.

6. Categorization of hospital emergency services must take a dynamic approach to manpower availability. A community hospital with well-trained, experienced emergency physicians backed by competent and available surgeons, internists, operating room personnel, and intensive care unit nurses (with or without house staff) has an emergency care capability that may compare favorably to emergency care resources in many university medical centers.

7. The university hospital should help evaluate the fiscal implications of categorization of hospital emergency services. (Publication's Abstract)

472. Boyd, David R., et al. "Categorization of Hospital Emergency Medical Capabilities in Illinois: A Statewide Experience." Illinois Medical Journal 146 (July 1974): 33-38.

The implementation of hospital categorization in Illinois is presented and the area-wide and regional medical planning process is outlined. Important steps in Illinois include legislation for categorization which allows hospitals to self-categorize and implementation of the Trauma Center concept which stresses regionalization of the emergency facilities in the state based on the categorization of hospital emergency services. Success of the program is attributed to the "classification of treatment centers based on a hospital's care capability and the distribution of selected trauma patients by the seriousness of their injuries," which indicates basic area-wide triage. Categorization guidelines for Illinois are presented as well as the EMS area-wide planning structure.

473. Cross, Ralph E., Jr. "Utilization Patterns in a Categorization System: Are the Concerns Real or Imagined?" JACEP 8 (July 1979): 284-86.

The author puts forward the concept that a well-planned emergency department categorization system will bring forth an orderly emergency medical care system and will provide the most effective use of qualified manpower and emergency department facilities.

474. Ford, J. Daniel. "Planning Depends on Analysis of Capabilities." Hospitals 47 (16 May 1973): 125-29.

The approach in the Chicago area for improvement of emergency medical service began with a thorough study of needs and an agreement to base change on the findings of the study. The next step was the organization of a permanent coordinating mechanism—the Emergency Medical Services Commission. Community health planning organizations are involved in the planning and implementation process through the activities of their area-wide EMS committees. This cooperative planning effort for emergency medical services promises to stimulate future cooperation among these hospital groups.

Literature

475. Forkosh, David S. "A Plan for the Organization of Emergency Services on Chicago's North Side." Illinois Medical Journal 142 (September 1977): 209-12.

> This is a report of the first area-wide EMS plan with categorization of hospital emergency capability in Illinois. The plan was completed by the Chicago North Side Commission on Health Planning, an agency composed of representatives from the fourteen member hospitals, consumers, and consumer representatives. A method of staff categorization in which each hospital categorized itself (subject to commission review) was used. The paper discusses interhospital transfers, a nursing education program for emergency room nursing personnel, psychiatric emergencies, and how the program integrated with the state trauma network, ambulance service, and community education. The general approach taken by this area-wide agency became the model for many other areas in Illinois.

476. Gibson, Geoffrey. "Categorization of Hospital Emergency Capabilities: Some Empirical Methods to Evaluate Appropriateness of Emergency Department Utilization." Journal of Trauma 18 (February 1978): 94-102.

> This paper posits a methodology and set of measures to assess appropriateness of utilization. The measures include: (1) distribution of ambulance and critically ill patients by AMA category of hospital; (2) utilization, characterized as a system under- or over-response or as appropriate utilization; and (3) physician judgments as to alternative treatment sites.

477. _____. "Measures of Appropriateness of Hospital Emergency Department Utilization." Paper presented at the American Public Health Association, San Francisco, November 1973. 27 p.

> Categorization is the method currently recommended and used by almost all emergency medical services agencies to match patient needs with resources for care. The method involves a survey of hospital emergency resources and categorizing, using a set of definitions and criteria developed by the American Medical Association. The author presents alternative methods of assessing emergency department utilization which expand upon the categorization approach by collecting additional data with minimum resources and maximum value for planning purposes.

478. Governor's Emergency Medical Services Advisory Council. Facility Task Force. State of Iowa. Report on a Program to Categorize Emergency Medical Service Facilities in Iowa Hospitals. Des Moines: February 1974. 157 p.

> The Facilities Task Force presents a study of regional categorization for all Iowa hospitals and develops a methodology which may prove useful to those in other areas. The report outlines the procedures prior to setting four classifications

Literature

of emergency services, including the assumptions underlying the need for categorization, the objectives and action taken to achieve the objectives and the recommendations of the Task Force.

479. Hampton, Oscar P., Jr. "Categorization of a Community's Hospital Emergency Services." Emergency Medicine Today 1 (April 1972): 1-8.

480. _____. "Categorization of Hospital Emergency Capabilities: A Progress Report." Emergency Medicine Today 4 (March 1975): 1-8.

481. _____. "Categorization of Hospital Emergency Capabilities: A Progress Report." American College of Surgeons Bulletin 60 (July 1975): 6-11.

482. _____. "A Rating System for Emergency Departments." Prism 2 (July 1974): 54-56.

> The author responds to the most significant criticisms of the AMA standards for categorization and indicates where revisions should be made. Progress to date toward categorization is reported as "not disappointing, but not very encouraging." The AMA guidelines are the best available and can be revised and updated, utilizing input from those in the field. The author encourages planners to move ahead with categorization while it can still be implemented by the private sector.

483. Harvey, John Collins. "Categorization of Emergency Capabilities." Hospitals 47 (16 May 1974): 69-72.

> Among the problems which confront a community desiring to implement categorization is the impact each facility may expect on its medical staff, on the number and type of professionals needed, and on its economic status due to payment characteristics of emergency department patients, and the number of admissions generated by the emergency department. There are potential benefits in a categorization which can be realized through a concerted effort in community and regional planning and in education for understanding and implementation.

484. Horty, John F. "Categorization: A Legal View." Hospitals 47 (16 May 1973): 75-80.

> Categorization is examined from a legal standpoint, outlining the areas of liability for emergency departments in cases where the patient did not receive the needed definitive care due to the failure of hospital personnel to respond adequately to the emergency. Categorization could furnish some legal protection and could be useful if the effect is to limit legally the emergency care of some hospitals beyond a specified level of sophistication. This determination must be given the force of state law and hospitals must be obligated to meet

every requirement for their own category. Although there
has been to date no legal test of categorization, the general
public must be carefully educated and prepared for it and
the specialized quality of care which it represents.

485. Kansas City. Area Hospital Association. Categorization of Emergency
Services. Kansas City, Mo.: 1974. 48 p.

This report documents results of a study to determine the
EMS capability of hospitals and other emergency service
agencies in the metropolitan Kansas City area. Four categories of emergency capabilities were adopted for this study:
(1) major emergency service, (2) emergency service, (3)
limited emergency service, and (4) no emergency service.

486. Klippel, Allen P. "Status Categorization is Dynamic." Hospitals 49
(16 July 1975): 151-52.

Based on the argument that rigid guidelines, such as those
embodied in the AMA emergency medical services categorization, may not be the best means of defining the emergency
capabilities of individual hospitals, a more flexible system
of categorization is suggested which would take into consideration each hospital's special care capabilities and capacities. Rather than being predicated largely on the capacity for handling major trauma patients late at night, the
new categorization would take into consideration all of the
facilities of each hospital at different hours of the day and
night, thereby helping to identify emergency resources more
realistically and to resolve conflicts inherent in the AMA
categorization.

487. Landau, Thomas. "Considerations of Regionalization and Categorization
in Hospital Emergency Planning." Master's thesis, MIT, Department
of Urban Studies and Planning, February 1975. 139 p.

This thesis explores some of the planning considerations
associated with hospital categorization and the need for a
regional plan of cooperation among hospitals. The fact
that the costs of high quality, specialized definitive care
are very high makes it imperative to consider the effectiveness
and efficiency of a categorization scheme. The model for
categorization introduced in the thesis develops a spatial
arrangement of emergency facilities which takes into account
epidemiological factors and the relative importance of stabilization and life support care. It is termed the horizontal
approach. It segments hospitals according to their care
capabilities in each of several diagnostic categories including trauma, coronary, high risk neonatal and pediatric,
psychiatric, poison, alcohol, and drug abuse. It takes into
account that the conflicting requirements for efficiency, accessibility, and quality of care may vary according to the
epidemiology of a particular type of emergency. Data requirements are presented for measuring emergency medical
coverage within a region and are computed and applied in
the model.

Literature

488. Mayberry, J.P., and Krass, M.E. "Autocategorization: A New Technique for Statistical Comparisons of Medical Diagnosis." JACEP 7 (June 1978): 237-40.

   Autocategorization is a new technique appropriate for studies involving relative frequencies of illness diagnoses using the International Classification of Diseases (U.S. Department of Health, Education, and Welfare, 1963). It is ideally suited for emergency department illness patterns. The technique uses the standard chi-square statistical test, but is novel in objectively determining the aggregation of diseases into categories for analysis. The numbers of observed occurrences of the various diseases are used, without applying any a priori judgments, to decide whether a disease should be analyzed alone, or aggregated with others. This technique, because it is based on the ICDA code, will permit comparisons of various studies while retaining the statistical validity of the individual studies.

489. Perrine, Edward L., and Bolt, W. David. Categorization of Emergency Room Facilities in Northeastern Kentucky. Morehead: Health Development Association of Northeastern Kentucky, 1973. 83 p.

   The purpose of the report is to present results of a survey of emergency room facilities in northeastern Kentucky, categorize those facilities according to American Medical Association criteria, and provide some suggestions for improvement. The survey of emergency room facilities covered a fifteen-county, primarily rural, region of northeastern Kentucky. The report discusses the reasons for increasing demand for use of EMS facilities, the methods used for collecting data, and the criteria used for categorizing the facilities. Various demographic data are presented to describe the region and its medical services.

490. Redmond, James M. "Categorization of Hospital Emergency Capabilities." Pennsylvania Medicine 78 (November 1975): 65-69.

   Categorization of medical emergency capabilities is a concept that has undergone a development process since it was first introduced. It offers the provider a technique to improve emergency medical services by identification of basic minimum requirements for life support, identification of specialized facilities for the care and treatment of the critically ill and injured, and the chance for close cooperative relationships among hospitals for the provision of a wide range of emergency medical services in a region.

491. Schnitker, Maurice A. "Categorization of Hospital Emergency Departments: How It Was Done in Ohio." Emergency Medicine Today 2 (January 1973): 1-6.

   The Community Council on Emergency Medical Care of Northwestern Ohio carried out a survey of all forty-two hospitals in the area. The emergency facility categories used were those developed by the National Academy of Sciences-National

Literature

Research Council with additional criteria formulated by the study team. Hospital categories were defined as (1) major, (2) basic, (3) standby, and (4) referral. The requirements for each category are detailed and programs which were made available for hospitals to self-improve are summarized.

492. Smith, J. Stanley. "Categorization: Matching Needs with Services." Pennsylvania Medicine 83 (September 1980): 33-34.

    Because most doctors and hospital administrators do not understand what is involved, they consider categorization a dirty word. The author explains the concept and why categorization is necessary. He also expands upon the function and work of categorization in the framework of the whole EMS system.

493. Tell, Robert. "Categorization: A Community Based Approach." JACEP 4 (March-April 1975): 152-55.

    This article deals with the community-based planning approach to categorization taken by Detroit. The author enumerates the problems which categorization presents to the community as well as to hospitals, and advocates communication among representatives of all components of the health care system in adopting categorization as an essential step in an effective emergency care system. Modification of the AMA guidelines and implementation of categorization in Detroit are summarized.

494. U.S. Department of Health, Education and Welfare. Division of Emergency Medical Services. Categorization of Emergency Medical Capabilities of Hospitals. Chicago: Categorization of Emergency Capabilities of Hospitals Symposium, September 9-10, 1975. 27 p.

    This paper is a technical assistance document and is a discussion of the role and importance of categorization of emergency facilities in planning and implementing sound and effective regional EMS systems to qualify for federal grant support under the Emergency Medical Services Systems Act of 1973 (PL 93-154). This working paper is intended to provide technical assistance to all grantees and potential grantees in their effort to develop EMS service systems for their respective locales. Emphasis in this draft paper is on the clinical rationale; patient impact; introduction of concepts and definitions; federal (DHEW) requirements; historic perspective; national progress and developmental models; exposure to methodologies; public education; economic issues; and legal ramifications. Also, a description of the interrelationship of the three associated EMS Act congressionally mandated components of facilities, critical care, and transfer of patients in the development of a comprehensive categorization program is discussed.

495. Waller, Julian A. "Categorizing Hospital Emergency Departments in Rural Areas." Clinical Medicine 82 (February 1975): 44-47.

Literature

This paper is concerned with one aspect of the treatment of schizophrenia, that is, the split personality that has characterized hospital emergency departments for the past quarter of a century. The emergency department is the major--in fact, the only--resource in the community for the prompt treatment of serious injury or illness. Simultaneously it has become the purveyor of outpatient care to a substantial segment of the population for a wide range of less serious emergency problems. Categorization deals only with the former and more traditional of these functions. (Publication's Abstract)

496. _____. "A Rural EMS Categorization System." Hospitals 48 (1 October 1974): 111-12, 114,116.

Waller reports that in a rural state such as Vermont, the AMA categorization system must be modified to (1) enable all hospitals to achieve minimum capability as a basic emergency department, and (2) categorize hospitals by performance criteria instead of the AMA staffing patterns. Criteria for basic emergency services are outlined and the planning which took place to develop and implement the system is discussed.

497. Waltz, Robert C. "Improving Emergency Medical Services in Ohio." Ohio State Medical Journal 70 (February 1974): 72-76.

This article outlines the requirements of EMS legislation (PL 93-154) which provide for creation of comprehensive emergency medical service systems throughout the country. Among the requirements is categorization of hospital facilities. This development was accomplished in Cleveland through a combined effort of the EMS council, medical society, and hospital association using guidelines established by the Academy of Medicine in Cleveland. Categories are: (1) major emergency care center; (2) general emergency care hospital; (3) basic emergency care hospital; and (4) resuscitation and referral facility.

498. Willemain, Thomas R. "A Coverage Model of Emergency Facility Categorization." JACEP 6 (March 1977): 89-93.

For any given type and severity of emergency, all hospitals in a region are divided into two classes: "definitive care facilities" and "stabilization facilities." A mathematical model is used to address the issue of the most appropriate mix of these two facility types where appropriateness is measured by the spatial coverage provided by the facility mix per dollar of system cost. Stabilization facilities are described by their cost and coverage relative to definitive care facilities. Conditions are specified on these parameters under which it is preferable, from the perspective of coverage per dollar, that all facilities offer definitive care. These criteria depend on the overall spatial density of facilities and the mode of patient access; assigning many facilities to a stabilization role is hardest to justify when there are relatively few facilities and patients tend to enter the system at the nearest facility. (Publication's Abstract)

Literature

499. Willemain, Thomas R., and Michaels, Harvey G. Coverage Models of Emergency Facilities Categorization. Cambridge: MIT, Innovative Resource Planning in Urban Public Safety Systems, June 1975. 45 p.

> Categorization of emergency facilities is meant to improve the match of clinical needs to level of services received, to improve spatial access to care and to reduce the cost of serving a region. For any given type and severity of emergency, facilities can be divided into two groups: definitive care facilities and stabilization facilities. Stabilization facilities are characterized by their relative cost and the extent to which they reduce the risk of travel to definitive care. Mathematical models of facilities located randomly in an infinite plane are used to address the critical planning issue of the appropriate number of each type of facility.

500. Youmans, Roger L., and Brose, Richard A. "A Basis for Classifying Hospital Emergency Services." Journal of the American Medical Association 213 (7 September 1970): 1647-51.

> This study, completed in the Kansas City metropolitan area, advocates a community-wide approach to categorization. Principles are presented for establishing continuity of care and specifying quality of care. All twenty-eight hospitals providing emergency care were surveyed using a point system of numerical values which were assigned to various essential aspects of emergency care delivery. Certain standards were specified, corresponding roughly to the guidelines of the American Society of Anesthesiology and the National Academy of Sciences, Committee on Emergency Rooms. Three classifications of emergency services were defined and called: major emergency facilities, emergency facilities, and provisional emergency facilities.

Utilization

501. Agisim, Elliot, and Woll, Myra. Wisconsin Emergency Department Utilization Study. Madison, Wis.: Department of Health and Social Services, March 1973. 39 p. (NTIS HRP 0003716)

> Data are presented from an emergency department utilization study initiated by the Wisconsin Emergency Medical Services Program to evaluate demands placed on the emergency medical services system in the state. The following characteristics of emergency department visits were assessed: incidence of selected diseases; urgency of visits; disposition of cases; method of transportation; and time and day of visits.

502. American Hospital Association. Emergency Services: The Hospital Emergency Department in an Emergency Care System. Chicago: 1972. 103 p.

> General principles for evaluating and planning the various elements of an emergency department and for establishing suitable policies and procedures are presented. Regional planning goals and objectives and their implementation are

Literature

considered, as is the problem of increased use of emergency departments for nonemergency uses. Community-wide planning for emergency services is discussed. Steps involved in developing an emergency department are delineated.

503. Areawide and Local Planning for Health Action. <u>Emergency Room Utilization in Central New York.</u> Syracuse: Ambulatory Care Committee, 1974. 74 p. (NTIS HRP 0004569)

> This document presents the findings of a utilization study of twelve emergency departments in a six-county area of central New York state. The main conclusion of the study is that nonurgent use of emergency departments should be reduced, and use of ambulatory care facilities should be increased.

504. Bobo, Timothy, et al. <u>Emergency Room Utilization: Overview and Implications.</u> Syracuse: Areawide and Local Planning for Health Action, December 1972. 25 p. (NTIS HRP 0009410)

> Emergency department utilization in the United States is reviewed, with emphasis on three utilization studies which were conducted in the Oswego and Lee Memorial Hospitals in Oswego County, New York; Tompkins County Hospital in New York; and three hospitals in Syracuse, New York. National and regional emergency room utilization trends are reviewed, and reasons for increased usage are given.

505. Bobzien, William, III. "The Observation-Holding Area: A Prospective Study." JACEP 8 (December 1979): 508-12.

> Although emergency department observation-holding units have been shown to be effective in limiting hospitalizations and improving the accuracy of disposition, the possibility of adverse outcome following discharge from such units has not been addressed. To establish the safety of the unit, a five-month prospective study of all patients admitted to this area was carried out and included long-term follow-up. 442 patients were admitted. Of these, 78 percent were improved upon discharge. Complications in the unit were minimal and there were no deaths. Long-term follow-up revealed four deaths (1 percent) and four patients (1 percent) who had complicated hospitalizations. Diagnosis, age, patient condition, and time of admission to the unit were predictive of the need for inpatient hospitalization. We conclude that the observation-holding unit, with appropriate supervision, represents a safe alternative disposition for selected emergency patients. (Author's Abstract)

506. Bureau of Health Planning and Resource Development. <u>Guidelines to Functional Programing, Equipping, and Designing Hospital Outpatient and Emergency Activities.</u> Bethesda, Md.: 1977. 217 p. (NTIS HRP-0017045)

Literature

Functional programing of outpatient and emergency activities of hospitals and various options for equipping and designing such facilities are outlined. The programing section presented an in-depth treatment of the subject through the use of a checklist and a pro forma example.

507. Burney, Richard E., and Sadler, Alfred M. "Resources Utilized for the Care of Surgical Patients in the Emergency Department." Medical Care 13 (December 1975): 1021-32.

    An approach to describing the medical problems and medical care rendered to surgical patients at an urban hospital's emergency department is explored. The study took place at the Yale-New Haven Medical Center in New Haven, Connecticut. A patient management classification system was developed and included five classes of surgical patients: (1) uncomplicated open wound, (2) uncomplicated closed injury, (3) major trauma, (4) visceral problems, and (5) chronic complaint. Quantitative estimates of the workload for all diagnostic and therapeutic services available to the emergency department patient were used in the development of a resources index.

508. Center for Hospital Management Engineering. A Study of Emergency Room Utilization. Chicago: 1975. 225 p.

    This report assesses the utilization of an emergency department. The main aim was to discover and analyze specific problems and to forward recommendations that will help to maximize the availability, adequacy, and accessibility of emergency rooms.

509. Chipman, Martin, et al. "Triage of Mass Casualties: Concepts for Coping with Mixed Battlefield Injuries." Military Medicine 145 (February 1980): 99-100.

    Triage application to mass disaster is presented. The basic requirements for good triage are: (1) preplanning; (2) full use of all available personnel; (3) forward movement of casualties with continuing triage at each medical echelon; and (4) simplicity.

510. Comprehensive Health Planning Council of South Florida. Goals and Guidelines for a System of Emergency Facilities for Dade County. Miami: June 1974. 29 p. (NTIS HRP-0007428)

    Presented are guidelines and criteria for emergency medical services and facilities in Dade County, Florida. Specific criteria are defined for four levels of emergency capability (categories). For each level, criteria are recommended in the areas of: emergency facility status, staffing, hospital support capability, equipment, communications, patient care, financial aspects, disaster plan, and evaluation.

Literature

511. Cowan, George S.M., et al. "The MUST Unit as a Combat Support Hospital: An Update Based Upon Recent Field Experience." Military Medicine 145 (February 1980): 117-20.

   The U.S. Army Medical Unit Self-Contained Transportable (MUST) Hospital, developed in 1963 and first deployed in Southeast Asia, is reevaluated from an operational and physical viewpoint.

512. Cram, A.E., and Tye, J.B. "Emergency Medical Services in Iowa." Journal of the Iowa Medical Society 68 (March 1978): 87-89.

   This paper summarizes steps being taken to upgrade emergency medical services in Iowa. Like police and fire services, the provision of prehospital emergency care is a public responsibility. Iowa physicians are challenged to participate actively in planning and implementing emergency medical services.

513. Davison, Stephen M. "Understanding the Growth of Emergency Department Utilization." Medical Care 16 (February 1978): 122-32.

   The author is not satisfied with the results of the research on utilization in the last fifteen years and tries to find a new approach outside the standard slant on demographic factors. He proposes the study of enabling and illness factors to find out the true reasons of emergency department utilization.

514. "Emergency Departments and the Non-Emergency Deluge." Medical World News 11 (December 1970): 23-28.

   Problems arising from the use of emergency departments (EDs) as a physician's office or ambulatory care facility are discussed in the context of Chicago's Cook County Hospital, and Cook County Hospital procedures are compared with activities of other county hospitals. The main impetus for the increasing use of EDs as the point of entry into the health care system has been failure in other aspects of the system such as lack of physicians and clinic facilities.

515. Fernández-Caballero, Carlos, et al. "The Spanish Speaking Patient and the EMS System." Emergency Medical Services 7 (July-August 1978): 57-59, 91.

   An underutilization of the EMS system by the Spanish-speaking minority appears to stem largely from language and cultural barriers. This problem has attracted minimum investigation and even fewer attempts at workable solutions. This paper reviewed the problem and offers some feasible recommendations for solutions.

516. Fletcher, J.R.,and Delfasse, C. "Computer Model for Simulation of Emergency Medical System." Military Medicine 144 (April 1979): 231-35.

Literature

A computer model has been developed which can be utilized in determining the resource requirements for optimal functioning of any emergency medical system.

517. Fraser, Claire L. "The Emergency Room: Its Use and Abuse." Master's thesis, Xavier University, Cincinnati, 1976. 73 p.

    This thesis studies the general characteristics of the patients using the emergency department at St. Mary's Hospital in Waterbury, Connecticut. Among the reasons cited by the author for the increased utilization of the ED are: shifts in population trends; nature of the community, and third-party payment. There is also a list of suggestions to improve utilization of the ED.

518. Fries, Brant E., et al. "Emergency Room Utilization: Data Reconstruction Using a Deterministic Simulation Model." Computer and Biomedical Research 10 (April 1977): 153-63.

    This is a study of the organization of the Emergency Department of Presbyterian Hospital, New York City. A SIMSCRIPT computer program was written to simulate the organization of the facility in order to reconstruct specialized and general treatment of patients. The method permits further evaluation by stochastic or deterministic simulation.

519. Gavette, J. William, and Thurber, Christine. Study of Three Small Upstate Emergency Departments. Rochester, N.Y.: Rochester Regional Medical Program, April 1972. 47 p. (NTIS HRP 0001655)

    This report presents statistics relating to the utilization of three rural community hospital emergency departments in New York. Results indicate using the services of a physician extender in the emergency room. The data show that the emergency department services a significant number of minor visits that might be effectively managed by a nurse practitioner. Full-time support of such a person on a three-shift basis could not be economically justified because of the low rate of visits to the department. It is suggested that the solution to the emergency department problem includes minimizing the demand for physician services, possibly by expanding service through a "convenience clinic."

520. Gibson, Geoffrey. "The Emergency Department as a Screening Point for Hospital Specialty Services: Inclusionary vs. Exclusionary Strategies." Social Science and Medicine 13A (June 1979): 495-98.

    This paper discusses two screening variations, inclusionary and exclusionary. Under the inclusionary strategy, the emergency department refers a substantial number of patients who should have been discharged from the emergency room to specialty clinics-units. Under the exclusionary strategy, the opposite occurs. The causes and consequences of the adoption of these strategies, or variations thereof, are also described.

Literature

521. Gibson, Geoffrey, and Gahn, Donald. "Health Services Research as a Management Tool in the Emergency Department." JACEP 5 (January 1976): 40-42.

> Researchers at Johns Hopkins University School of Medicine, with a grant under section 1205 of the Emergency Medical Services Systems (EMSS) Act of 1973 from the National Center for Health Services Research (DHEW), are doing three research projects pertaining to the quality and effectiveness of care and management in the emergency department. Project 1 concerns assessing the impact of categorization of facilities and ambulance and communications improvements on the use of emergency departments and ambulances. Project 2 assesses the impact of triage nursing, patient exit interviews, patient advocacy, nursing audit, walk-in clinics, and education of asthmatic patients on emergency department care. Project 3 investigates the effect of specific clinical procedures on patient outcome. (Publication's Abstract)

522. Gold, Marsha R., and Rosenberg, Robert G. "Use of Emergency Room Services by the Population of a Neighborhood Health Center." Health Services Report 89 (January-February 1974): 65-70.

> Utilization of the emergency department of the Children's Hospital Medical Center and the Martha Eliot Health Center in Boston, Massachusetts, is investigated. Children residing in the target area were surveyed in an attempt to determine the extent to which each center was used, what variables determined differences in such use, and the extent to which both centers were used by the same children and which different patterns of use could be isolated.

523. Graves, Harris B. "ACEP Surveys Hospital Triage Systems." JACEP 1 (November-December 1972): 31-33.

> This is a study of forty community hospitals of more than two hundred beds in order to evaluate their triage systems. The hospitals ranged up to eleven-hundred beds. Their emergency department patient load ranged from 15,000 to 150,000 patients per year.

524. Gray, Lois, and Godley, Carol. Emergency Medical Services and Neighborhood Health Centers. 2 vols. Washington, D.C.: National Association of Neighborhood Health Centers, August 1975. Vol. 1, 163 p; vol. 2, 93 p. (NTIS PB 262 632/633)

> The research developed a methodology to investigate and describe the availability and utilization of emergency medical services in federally supported neighborhood health centers. This information is pertinent to the assessment of the impact of NHC emergency services on target populations being served and an assessment of NHC emergency medical services' role in the overall spectrum of health and medical care. This report accomplished all objectives satisfactorily.

Literature

525. Hannan, Edward. "Planning an Emergency Department Holding Unit." Socio-Economic Planning Sciences 9 (October 1975): 179-88.

   A computer simulation model of the queuing process in an emergency department holding unit is presented. The model developed to evaluate the effects of changes in demand and utilization policies upon congestion in the unit. Bed utilization percentages, census level, and daily service level criteria are used to measure congestion.

526. Huffine, Carol L., and Craig, Thomas J. "Social Factors in the Utilization of an Urban Psychiatric Emergency Service." Archives of General Psychiatry 30 (February 1974): 249-55.

   Demographical and institutional factors affecting the utilization of a twenty-four hour psychiatric emergency service for adults and adolescents at Johns Hopkins Hospital, Baltimore, are analyzed in a study of 270 users of the service during July and August 1971. Characteristics of patients and the areas in which they reside are described, with special attention to the social characteristics found to be associated with high admission rates. Based on the study findings, suggestions are offered of ways in which services might be altered to meet the treatment needs of inner-city populations more effectively.

527. Jacobs, Arthur R., et al. "Emergency Department Utilization in an Urban Community: Implications for Community Ambulatory Care." Journal of the American Medical Association 216 (April 1971): 307-12.

   This article analyzes the use of hospital emergency departments in Rochester, New York, in 1968, and discusses their use for ambulatory care in the region. A random sample of emergency department cases was drawn from the records of all nine area hospitals to obtain data. It was found that the number of visits to hospital emergency departments had increased five times faster than the general population of the area over the previous decade.

528. Jonas, Steven, et al. "Monitoring Utilization of a Municipal Emergency Department." Hospital Topics 54 (January-February 1976): 43-48.

   This is a report of a study conducted at Morrisania City Hospital, Bronx, New York, to develop method for collecting data on emergency department utilization and users' characteristics.

529. Jones, Susan L., et al. "Identification of Patients in Need of Psychiatric Intervention Visiting an Emergency Facility." Medical Care 16 (May 1978): 372-82.

   The utilization of the emergency room at a small community hospital located in a black inner-city area is investigated. Patients are classified according to a criterion for psychiatric intervention for the purpose of making staffing pattern recommendations. Psychiatric patients and nonpsychiatric

Literature

patients are classified by age, marital status, previous admissions to the ER, time of arrival and time spent in the ER, and circumstances of mode of arrival in the ER. The criterion of psychiatric intervention is viewed as providing an additional dimension in the study of the emergency room, a hospital service which is providing increasing routine and nonroutine medical care to the general population.

530. Kanwit, John H., and Gettinger, C. Earl. <u>Hospital Emergency Services in Vermont.</u> Burlington, Vt.: State Department of Health, August 1971. 58 p. (NTIS HRP-0002346)

    Results of on-site observation and interviews covering twenty-one hospitals providing emergency department service to Vermont patients are reported. The purpose of the survey was to document those services provided by emergency departments with respect to facilities, staffing, and scope of care. Most of the departments were found to be small, but to contain fairly comprehensive laboratory facilities and stores of blood types. Some had the capacity to handle only one or two patients at the same time. Often, the hospital and the emergency room were difficult to find due to lack of directional signs. Greatest difficulty was shown to be in maintaining immediately available staff.

531. Karas, Stephen, Jr. "Cyclicality of Hospital Admissions and Emergency Department Visits." JACEP 4 (March-April 1975): 126-28.

    This study at the Los Angeles County-University of Southern California Medical Center developed a method of cyclical analysis of ED utilization. The high peak occurred on Mondays and Tuesdays, and the low on Saturdays and Sundays.

532. Kelman, Howard R., and Lane, Dorothy. <u>Irreducible Functions of the Hospital Emergency Room.</u> Stony Brook: State University of New York, Health Sciences Center, November 1975. 42 p.

    During the last two decades the purposes and problems of the hospital emergency department have been of critical concern both in terms of continually increasing demands for nonurgent care from populations believed lacking primary care alternatives, and more recently in upgrading the capacity of the emergency department to respond to needs of urgent life-threatening injuries and illness. The results of a recently conducted study have been analyzed in an attempt to forecast and define a more rational role for a community hospital emergency room, typically located in a suburban area experiencing rapid population growth without commensurate increase in primary care resources.

533. Kresojevich, Ralph, et al. "The Emergency Department Groupy." JACEP 3 (March-April 1974): 81-84.

    Twenty-nine patients who were viewed as chronically misusing the services of the Detroit General Hospital Emergency de-

Literature

partment were identified by the triage nurse, interviewed, and their medical records reviewed. They accounted for less than 2 percent of all patient visits, far less than the emergency department personnel had estimated. These patients engendered a strong emotional response in department personnel and evinced the ability to raze professional barriers. As this capability is shared with the "groupy" who haunts rock groups, such a patient was dubbed an "emergency department groupy." The groupies were best characterized by their abnormally high visit frequency, as many as thirty-one in a year, with an average of eleven. Men tended to make more visits than women. Groupies could not be distinguished on the basis of sex or race. However, they were older, poorer, and more socially isolated than other patients. Their number included an increased percentage of people with alcoholic problems. (Publication's Abstract)

534. Krome, Ronald L., et al. "A Study of Emergency Medical Services in the Detroit Metropolitan Area." JACEP 2 (May-June 1973): 177-83.

Emergency facilities in the Detroit metropolitan area were studied in 1970 utilizing questionnaires and on-site surveys. This article reports on the procedures and results of the study. Only one hospital provided totally comprehensive emergency services while 25 percent could provide little more than first aid. Most (66 percent) could offer routine emergency care but would have to transfer patients with major problems. It was found that the admission policy of the hospital, often unidentified in such surveys, may play a pivotal role in the achievement of high quality emergency patient care.

535. Kvalseth, Tarald O., and Deems, John M. "Statistical Models of the Demand for Emergency Medical Services in an Urban Area." American Journal of Public Health 69 (March 1979): 250-55.

Statistical models are presented for the emergency medical services demand in an urban area as it relates to various socioeconomic, demographic, and other characteristics of the area. Individual models were prepared for different types of medical emergencies. The site studied was Atlanta.

536. Landers, Gary A., et al. "Observation Ward Utilization." JACEP 4 (March-April 1975): 123-25.

The policies, staffing, and procedures of the Kansas City General Hospital and Medical Center, observation ward in the emergency department, are the aims of this study. One of the findings stresses the importance of the observation ward in the operation of the emergency department.

537. Larsen, Kenneth T., et al. "Triage: A Logical Algorithmic Alternative to a Non-System." JACEP 2 (May-June 1973): 183-87.

Literature

This article reports the experience at DeWitt Army Hospital, Fort Belvoir, Virginia, where an algorithm was implemented to perform the triage function.

538. LeTourneau, Barbara, et al. "Critical Care in an Emergency Department." Annals of Emergency Medicine 9 (March 1980): 126-30.

   The article deals with a one-year review of resuscitation in the emergency department at Hennepin County Medical Center, Minneapolis.

539. Lohrisch, David Niven. "Systems Analysis of a Hospital Based Rural Emergency Medical Service System." Ph.D. dissertation, Mississippi University, August 1975. 129 p.

   A systems approach is used to analyze a hospital-based rural emergency medical service system. Introductory information on systems analysis is provided and a review of the literature on EMS evaluation utilization and systems analysis is included. In the analysis of a hospital-based rural EMS system, patients were selected who entered the emergency medical system of the Oxford-Lafayette County area of Mississippi.

540. Manning, Beatrice, and Singleton, Sharla. Emergency Room Utilization at Day Kimball Hospital: A Preliminary Report. Storrs: University of Connecticut, Department of Agricultural Economics and Rural Sociology, December 1976. 20 p.

   The authors report on the use of the emergency department at Day Kimball Hospital, Putman, Connecticut, a poor rural area. The study was intended to identify types of emergency department utilization, purposes of such usage, and patterns, if there were any.

541. Mannon, James M. "Time, Work and Decision-Making in Emergency Medicine: In a Hospital Emergency Room." Ph.D. dissertation, Southern Illinois University, 1975. 221 p.

   Mannon's goal was to discover the central problems faced by emergency department staff as they provide care to emergency department patients. He found that ED staff face three main problems: (1) the staff never knows when patients will arrive for treatment; (2) the staff could not predict when the more serious cases would arrive; and (3) the staff could neither control nor predict the number of patients who would demand treatment at any time.

542. Mattox, Kenneth L. "Public Entry Into Emergency Medical Services Systems." JACEP 5 (February 1976): 128-31.

   Emergency facilities and personnel are used for more non-emergency care than true emergency cases. Much of the public is not prepared to recognize an emergency situation, and does not know where to go for help. Some of the recommendations for improving public access to EMS systems are: a good communications system for triage and information, ambulatory centers for nonemergency care, and use of medical extenders.

543. Owens, Susan R., et al. Patterns of Utilization of the Emergency Room at Middlesex Memorial Hospital. Middletown: Midstate Connecticut River Estuary Comprehensive Health Planning Council, July 1973. 86 p.

This study examines structural variables of the health system, and social and demographic variables of patients using emergency departments in the area in question. Demographic characteristics of the subjects investigated include age, sex, race, employment status, occupation, education, socioeconomic status, payment mechanism, place of residence, and length of residence in the county. Findings indicate that emergency services are taking over some of the primary care functions in the community, and ED users are likely to be recent arrivals in the area, and of low socioeconomic status.

544. Plant, Janet, and Ames, Seth. "Emergency/Outpatient Satellites Serve as Rural Outposts." Hospitals 52 (1 March 1978): 878-902.

Several New Hampshire communities, faced with sudden population growth and difficulty in recruiting physicians, jointly developed combined emergency and outpatient satellite facilities. This paper discusses services, staffing, operations, financing, and impact.

545. Pozen, Michael W., et al. "The Usefulness of a Predictive Instrument to Reduce Inappropriate Admissions to the Coronary Care Unit." Annals of Internal Medicine 92 (Februrary 1980): 238-42.

A mathematical instrument was developed to supplement the diagnostic information available to physicians in the emergency room to improve physicians' diagnostic accuracy in managing patients with acute ischemic heart disease and thereby reducing inappropriate coronary care unit admissions. The instrument was empirically derived and is based on nine clinical, historical, and electrocardiographic predictive variables. Probabilities of acute ischemic heart disease generated by the instrument were given to the house staff in an emergency room during alternate months.

546. Region Three Health Planning Council. Interim Study of Fort Wayne, Indiana Hospital's Emergency Room Utilization. Fort Wayne, Ind.: March 1975. 12 p. (NTIS HRP-0003627)

Utilization patterns were evaluated with respect to primary diagnosis of disease or trauma, discharge status, age, sex, patient origination, and level of emergency. Seven variables were selected from all base period emergency department records. These included address, zip code, age, sex, disease, emergency level, and admission status. Criteria were developed for classifying an emergency department visit as a true emergency, a nonemergency, or an uncertain borderline case.

Literature

547. Rosen, Pet, et al. "A Method of Triage Within an Emergency Department." JACEP 3 (March-April 1974): 85-86.

> The University of Chicago emergency department developed a triage system composed of three categories: true emergency, urgent, and nonemergency.

548. Sandler, Alan P., and Chan, Linda S. "Mexican-American Folk Belief in a Pediatric Emergency Room." Medical Care 16 (September 1978): 778-84.

> The authors study the pattern, extent, and patient care implications of medical folk belief in the Mexican-American population using a pediatric emergency department in the Los Angeles County area. Folk belief is common among the population of Hispanic origin which utilizes this service. The illness for which care is sought, however, is felt to be amenable to scientific care and therefore medical folk belief is not often a clinically relevant factor in the emergency department setting.

549. Selby, Jones W., et al. "Sex Differences Among Clients of an Emergency Care Unit for Alcoholism." Journal of Clinical Psychology 34 (April 1978): 567-68.

> This paper compares males and females who visit the emergency department for treatment of alcohol-related crises. Among the characteristics studied are age, employment status, marital status, and educational level.

550. Shiver, J.M., et al. "Center Provides Emergency Care Without Unneeded Inpatient Units." Hospitals 53 (16 April 1979): 116-19.

> The Ambulatory Care Center-Emergency Services System (ACCESS) was established to provide immediate ambulatory and emergency care in Fairfax, Virginia, and, through referrals to Fairfax Hospital's emergency department, ensure more extensive emergency or in-patient care, as required.

551. Slay, Larry E., and Riskin, Wayne G. "Algorithm-Directed Triage in an Emergency Department." JACEP 5 (November 1976): 869-76.

> This article reports on the use of "screeners" to perform triage at Brooke Army Medical Center, Emergency Services Section. The triage is algorithm-directed. The screeners, medical corpsmen, have 25 hours of classroom and 120 hours of on-the-job training.

552. Steinmetz, Nicholas, and Hoey, John R. "Hospital Emergency Room Utilization in Montreal before and after Medicare. The Quebec Experience." Medical Care 16 (February 1978): 133-39.

> The authors study the impact of the introduction of Medicare in Quebec on emergency department utilization. Findings show that after Medicare, emergency department visits greatly increased.

Literature

553. Stratmann, William, and Ullman, Ralph. "Study of Consumer Attitudes About Health Care: The Role of the Emergency Room." <u>Medical Care</u> 13 (December 1975): 1033-43.

> A study of consumer attitudes was conducted to evaluate the utilization of emergency rooms for health care. Data were obtained from a community survey of households in the Rochester, New York, area. A survey questionnaire was developed to document the utilization of medical care facilities and to elicit from respondents the reasons for reported visits. The respondents also were asked about the urgency of any medical condition that necessitated emergency room visits. Contrary to the traditional role of the emergency room as a care source for the treatment of urgent medical needs, it was evident that a substantial number of people utilized the emergency room for nonurgent problems.

554. Thomas, J. William. <u>Emergency System Simulator (ESSIM): User's Guide</u>. Philadelphia: University of Pennsylvania, December 1974. 30 p.

> The Emergency System Simulator (ESSIM) is a simulation model that allows EMS planners to investigate the interdependencies among various elements comprising an EMS system. ESSIM addresses the following questions: (1) How should the region be structured in terms of ambulance service districts and emergency room catchment areas? (2) Is the number of emergency facilities and the resources within each adequate for the needs of the region? Could some emergency rooms be closed? (3) How should existing emergency facilities be categorized, and what is the impact of categorization on hospital admissions and bed-days? (4) Should ambulances be categorized, as facilities often are?

555. Thompson, C. Thomas, and Lewis, James E. "Emergency Medical Services as a Model for Rural Health Care Delivery." <u>Journal of the Oklahoma State Medical Association</u> 71 (January 1978): 26-29.

> This paper identifies the steps necessary to provide a voluntary, cooperative arrangement within which communities and hospitals can match their needs and capabilities so as to meet, at minimum, the emergency medical service needs of Oklahoma's small town and rural areas.

556. Ullman, Ralph, et al. "An Emergency Room's Patients: Their Characteristics and Utilization of Hospital Services." <u>Medical Care</u> 13 (December 1975): 1011-20.

> Utilization of the emergency room at an urban community hospital is studied in a format designed to accomplish three complementary objectives: (1) to characterize a sample of individual patients, rather than an unweighted sample of visits; (2) to estimate the number of individuals served during a specified period and the magnitude of the relationship between these patients and the utilization of other hospital services; and (3) to introduce the patient's "frequency-of-visit"

Literature

as an important variable in the analysis of emergency room utilization. Some specific findings are: (1) the vast majority of patients who used the emergency room did so very infrequently: 46,527 visits were made in one year by an estimated 34,286 different patients; (2) an estimated 2,586 patients made three or more visits during the year; a disproportionately large number of the "high-frequency" users were black, low-income, and from inner-city areas; a relatively small percentage of their visits were for accidental injury. (3) Approximately 53 percent of the hospitals inpatient admissions and 68 percent of the inpatient days were generated by patients who also made at least one emergency room visit during the year studied. (Publication's Abstract)

557. _____. "Impact of a Primary Care Group Practice on Emergency Room Utilization at a Community Hospital." Medical Care 16 (September 1978): 723-29.

This is a report on the study of the effects of a primary care group practice on the utilization of a community hospital emergency department. Findings seem to show that the primary care group practice effected a noticeable reduction in pediatric and adult emergency department use.

558. Vaughn, Byon, et al. "Effective Algorithm-Based Triage and Self-Care Protocols: Quality Medicine at Lower Costs." Annals of Emergency Medicine 9 (January 1980): 31-36.

The triage phase of an algorithm-based medical care system was analyzed in three military environments. Combat medics triaged 4,799 patients using a physician-prepared triage manual which specified levels of initial health care based on the patient's presented complaints and a brief history. The study demonstrates that personnel receiving basic medical training and orientation to an algorithm-directed triage system can direct military patients to appropriate levels of health care.

559. Walker, Lynn Levi. "The Emergency Department--Entry Point Into the Health Care System." JACEP (March-April 1975): 129-32.

In order to find out about the role of the emergency department as an entry point into the health care system in a community general hospital, a study was done to assess: (1) the emergency department as a referral source of hospital inpatients, and (2) its effect upon the private practice of medicine in the community. The results indicate that the emergency department was not in competition with the private physician, and that it was a major source of hospital inpatients.

560. _____. "Emergency Room in a Community General Hospital: A Study of Characteristics, Attitudes, and Usage Patterns by Patients." Ph.D. dissertation, Oklahoma University, Oklahoma City, 1973. 164 p. (NTIS HRP-0010493)

A study of the emergency department of South Community Hospital, Oklahoma City, is presented. Factors and attitudes influencing utilization of the emergency department are examined in a comparison of inpatient and emergency department patient records and through interviews with patients, physicians, and nursing personnel. Study results are said to confirm that the emergency department was not being used for its intended purpose; the ratio among 662 patients was found to be one emergency to five urgent to three non-emergency cases. This clinic function is attributed to the point-of-entry problem in the urban health care system and to the inaccessibility of physicians after hours.

561. _____. "Inpatient and Emergency Department Utilization: The Effect of Distance, Social Class, Age, Sex, and Marital Status." JACEP 5 (February 1976): 105-10.

This article reports on a study done to attempt to evaluate whether patients utilizing the inpatient facilities and the emergency department of two hospitals were representative of the population. The experiment wanted to confirm the premises that if patient demands were uniform and there were no barriers to emergency department utilization, (1) emergency patients would be a demographical representation of the hospital geographical area, and (2) factors such as age, sex, marital status, and social class, would be relatively uniform between inpatients and emergency department patients.

562. Walker, Lynn Levi, and Miller, Sheldon I. "Sensitivity to Symptoms in Patients Utilizing an Emergency Department." JACEP 2 (September-October 1973): 321-26.

To evaluate the concern that nonemergent patients are inappropriately crowding emergency facilities, the level of sensitivity to a list of symptoms was determined for 522 patients utilizing an emergency department. Patients selected those symptoms they regarded sufficiently serious to warrant medical consultation. Using the attitudinal scale of Hetherington and Hopkins, the selections permitted classifying patients into one of three groups: hypersensitive, sensitive, and insensitive. Sensitive patients appropriately recognized the medical significance of symptoms. Insensitive patients thought serious symptoms were trivial while hypersensitive patients felt trivial symptoms were serious. The majority, 55 percent, were found symptom insensitive. Only two were sensitive to symptoms. Relating the three categories to characteristics of the patient population, patients with non-emergent conditions, lower social class, and those without other physician contact were found more frequently symptom insensitive (i.e., less capable of properly identifying serious symptoms). (Publication's Abstract)

563. William, B.T. "Admission to Hospital and Day of the Week." Public Health 93 (May 1979): 173-76.

Literature

> The daily pattern of admission to a hospital over a period of one year is analyzed. Results show that emergency admissions peak early in the week, remained constant in midweek, and fell on weekends.

564. Wilson, Frank P., et al. "Algorithm-Directed Triage of Pediatric Patients: A Prospective Study." JAMA 243 (18 April 1980): 1528-31.

> This paper, citing the example of an army corpsman, demonstrates that individuals lacking formal medical training can successfully utilize physician-written triage algorithms to rate patients' need for care in emergency facilities.

565. Wingert, Willis, et al. "Influence of Family Organization on the Utilization of Pediatric Emergency Services." Pediatrics 4 (November 1968): 743-51.

> The influence of family organization on pediatric emergency service utilization is examined. Patterns of obtaining medical care for children from broken, lower socioeconomic families did not differ significantly from those of intact families. Many separated and divorced mothers handled their children's health problems adequately in spite of economic and transportation problems. Stability and presence of both parents were not synonymous. It is noted that the broken family may actually be quite stable due to hidden mates, guidance from appropriate social agencies, and social norms which assign medical nursing care to mothers.

E. CRITICAL CARE UNITS

This section requires providing access, including transportation, to specialized critical care units. These units should be the number and variety necessary to meet the demands of the service area and are to include: (1) "Trauma"; (2) "Burn Care"; (3) "Spinal Cord Injury"; (4) "Poisoning"; (5) "Acute Cardiac Care"; (6) "High Risk Infant"; and (7) "Behavioral Emergencies."

Trauma

Trauma is the most common and complex emergent condition to which the EMS system will respond. Based upon an identification of patients by trauma diagnosis, special needs and magnitude of injury or illness, each EMS region should conceptualize and design a system of emergency care for prehospital, hospital, and interhospital and critical care phases. Facilities should be vertically designated according to the American College of Surgeons criteria for initial and definitive care.

566. Bailey, Judith A. "Development of a Regional Trauma Center: Nursing Approach." Nursing Clinics of North America 13 (June 1978): 255-65.

Literature

The Regional Trauma Center at University Hospital in San Diego was primarily developed and designed using nursing input. The nurse coordinator and clinical head nurse played a primary role in planning the unit. As a result, it has proved to be a workable and efficient facility supplied with modern and sophisticated equipment.

567. Bregande, Barbara J. "Design of Intensive Care Units." Hospital Topics 51 (October 1973): 41-42.

    Health care providers and architects pay a minimal amount of attention to program development of intensive care units (ICU). The basic requirements for an ICU are: the delivery of care to patients in individually identified spaces or units; emphasis on the preventative as well as restorative functions of intensive care rendered as opposed to a patient's critical condition; and optimum environmental conditions, including units equipped with assistive devices developed by the best modern medical technology.

568. Burns, C.M. "Symposium on Trauma for the General Surgeon. 1. An Accident Health Care Program: The Organization and Development of Regional Trauma Units." Canadian Journal of Surgery 21 (November 1978): 507-10.

    This paper recommends the development of a Canadian accident health care delivery and audit system which would improve the health care standard and provide a data base for the implementation of effective accident prevention campaigns. Among the principal features of the system are radio-equipped ambulance stations situated between regional trauma units, and provincial trauma registries.

569. Cowley, R. Adams. "Trauma Center: A New Concept for the Delivery of Critical Care." Journal of the Medical Society of New Jersey 74 (November 1977): 979-87

    This article describes the functions of the Maryland Institute for Emergency Medicine. That unit provides total care to the trauma victim with multiple injuries. The trauma center is the hub of a system of emergency medical care, which also provides transportation, communication, referral centers, and education.

570. Cowley, R. Adams, and Scalan, Elizabeth. "University Trauma Center: Operation, Design and Staffing." American Surgeon 45 (February 1979): 79-85.

    This paper describes fifteen years' experience of the Maryland Institute for Emergency Medical Services (MIEMS). The authors believe that MIEMS can be considered a model for the design, staffing, and operation of a trauma center.

571. DeClaris, Nicholas, et al. "A Systems Approach to Intensive Care Medicine." American Surgeon 45 (February 1979): 86-92.

Literature

After a decade of practical experience, intensive care medicine proved it was successful in saving human lives. This article demonstrates that intensive care medicine, in order to be useful, needs a system approach and special facilities.

572. Felknor, Rhea. "Trauma Center: Reversing the Process of Dying." RN Magazine 37 (September 1974): 45-51.

    The Maryland Institute for Emergency Medicine, in downtown Baltimore, is not just another operating room. The institute is unique for its concentration on treating trauma victims whose lives are imperiled by injury to more than one body system.

573. Fischer, Ronald P., et al. "Direct Transfer to Operating Room Improves Care of Trauma Patients: A Simple, Economically Feasible Plan for Large Hospitals." JAMA 240 (13 October 1978): 1731-32.

    This study, based on nine years' experience with approximately four thousand patients, reveals that the immediate conveyance of critically injured patients to the operating room, bypassing the emergency room, saves lives and reduces the burden on overcrowded emergency rooms.

574. Maddox, Darrell. "Community Hospital Gears Up to Provide Intensive Care." Modern Hospital 118 (January 1972): 100-102.

    The author relates the Anaheim, California, Memorial Hospital experience to develop an interdisciplinary acute care treatment unit with around-the-clock physician coverage.

575. Maull, Kimball I., and Haynes, B.W. "The Integrated Trauma Service Concept." JACEP 6 (November 1977): 497-99.

    The authors present the concept of integrated trauma service. This service is obtained through the coordination of pre-existing manpower and other resources to insure the availability of emergency medical care to patients in need of critical care treatment.

576. Moerkirk, George E., and Grottenthaler, Joel. "Trauma Systems: Pennsylvania's Progress and Challenge." Pennsylvania Medicine 83 (September 1980): 27-32.

    Pennsylvania's trauma system development and progress is presented. This trauma system must be considered within the context of a much larger EMS system.

577. More, G., and Sandler, R. Feasibility Analysis for a Consolidated Emergency Trauma Center. Ann Arbor, Mich.: CSF, 1973. 56 p.

    This study assesses the impact of a consolidated emergency trauma center at one of two specific hospitals. Some of the aspects studied were the surgical facilities, elective surgery, and finances. There was some increase in revenues in one of the units after the consolidation.

Literature

578. Mullner, Ross, and Goldberg, Jack. "The Illinois Trauma System: Changes in Patient Survival Patterns Following Vehicular Injuries." JACEP 6 (September 1977): 393-96.

   The impact of the Illinois Trauma Program on Region 5, Southern Illinois, was evaluated. This was done by comparing data referring to vehicular injuries and deaths for a four-year period: two years prior to the system implementation, 1970-71, and two years after the implementation, 1972-73. The results indicate that there was a significant decrease in mortality after the trauma system was initiated.

579. "Special Care Units Have Special Design Requirements." Modern Hospital 118 (March 1972): 105-7.

   A set of criteria was developed to help in the design of special care units: (1) locate the area close to ambulance entrance; (2) locate intensive care adjacent to beds to be used for progressive care; (3) create a restful and attractive environment; and (4) create a safe electrical environment.

580. A System Approach to the Care of the Trauma Victim. Grand Rapids, Mich.: EMS Patient Care Systems Planning and Implementation Symposia, November 11-13, 1975. 79 p.

   The purpose of this paper as related to a trauma patient care system is to develop important concepts of what constitutes an effective system of emergency medical care for critically injured trauma patients. It has been developed in ten chapters, bringing in and tying together into a systems approach all of the key elements that have heretofore been addressed and funded only in a fragmented, general categorical and uncoordinated manner.

581. Taylor, Blaine. "Close Encounters of the Cowley Kind: An Exclusive Journal Interview with R. Adams Cowley, MD, Director of the Maryland Institute for Emergency Medical Services, State of Maryland." Maryland State Medical Journal 27 (June 1978): 35-49.

   This is an interview with Dr. R. Adams Cowley, director of the Maryland Institute for Emergency Medical Services (MIEMS), Baltimore.

582. Teufel, William, and Trunkey, Donald D. "Trauma Centers: A Pragmatic Approach to Need, Cost, and Staffing Patterns." JACEP 6 (December 1977): 546-51.

   Based on the premise that the recommendations of the American College of Surgeons Committee on Trauma and the Health Services Administration are unrealistic in their dealing with staffing and cost of trauma center, the authors put forth their own recommendations for a practical approach to the management of a nonuniversity community hospital trauma unit.

Literature

583. Weil, Max Harry, and Shubin, Herbert. "Centers for the Critically Ill." Modern Medicine 39 (31 May 1971): 86-99.

> The development of specialty units is studied. Those units that exist in large hospitals--coronary care, cardiac care, respiratory care, shock, and renal dialysis--need to be monitored constantly. If there is a lack of adequate monitoring, there is threat to the survival of the patient.

584. Weston, P.A.M. "First-Line Medical Care for the Injured." Injury 4 (February 1973): 208-12.

> The development of a joint hospital and general practitioner organization in East Cumberland, England, to provide medical care to the seriously injured before they reach the hospital is described. The advantages of such a joint organization are presented.

Burn Care

Each EMS system or region should conceptualize and design a system of emergent care for the prehospital, hospital, interhospital, and critical care phases for major burn injury. Facilities should be designated for initial and definitive care based upon American Burn Association criteria.

585. Bobo, Phillip K. "Burn Care: Impact or Regionalization in Region Two--1978." Journal of the Medical Association of the State of Alabama 49 (November 1979): 14-16, 35-36, 46-47.

> A regional burn program, as part of a comprehensive EMS system, was developed in west Alabama during 1975 to 1978. This study supports the concept of improved care for victims of major burns through improved patient outcome, through identification and successive triage to a specially designed center for expert definitive care.

586. Brigham, Peter A., and DeClement, Frederic A. "Burn Care in Pennsylvania, 1980." Pennsylvania Medicine 83 (September 1980): 35-38.

> The development of the last ten years in treatment of the burn victim in Pennsylvania is presented. Main aspects covered are: referral regions and air transportation.

587. "Burn Patients Go Through Three Treatment Stages in This Unit." Modern Hospital 118 (January 1972): 93-95.

> The function of the burn center of University of Michigan Hospital, Ann Arbor, is described. This special care unit grew out of a smaller burn unit which was established at University Hospital in 1960. The center is divided into three main care areas: (1) the emergent stage; (2) the acute period; and (3) rehabilitative period.

Literature

588. Comprehensive Health Planning Council of Southwestern Indiana. <u>Analysis of Burn Care Services and Needs in Southwestern Indiana with Conclusions and Recommendations.</u> Evansville, Ind.: Community Health Services Committee, August 1974. 41 p. (NTIS HRP-0003237)

   The need for specialized burn care facilities in Health Region 13 of southwestern Indiana is assessed in a study of burn care services in the region. The results suggested that there were not enough burn patients to justify establishing a burn care service. Such units operate at a relatively high cost per patient and with low patient utilization.

589. Edlich, Richard F., et al. "Emergency Department Treatment, Triage and Transfer Protocols for the Burn Patient." JACEP 7 (April 1978): 152-58.

   Emergency department treatment, triage, and transfer protocols for patients with major thermal injury have been devised by the three burn centers in Virginia. A burn nurse educator has presented these guidelines to the emergency departments of Virginia. The development of these protocols has considerably improved the immediate care of the victims of thermal injury who are transferred to the burn centers in the Commonwealth of Virginia. (Author's Abstract)

590. Feck, Gerald, et al. "A Systems Model for Burn Care." <u>Medical Care</u> 18 (February 1980): 211-18.

   Demand for burn patient treatment was evaluated in fifty-seven counties in New York State. Findings show that existing planning formulae which were designed for events of common occurrence were found to project conditions of overflow and underutilization incompletely when applied to regional burn units. To correct this, objective planning models were designed especially for burn care centers.

591. Hayter, Jean. "Emergency Nursing Care of the Burned Patient." <u>Nursing Clinics of North America</u> 13 (June 1978): 223-34.

   In providing emergency nursing care to severely burned patients, lifesaving measures receive the highest priority. The patient's condition is quickly evaluated and then, fluid and electrolyte loss is estimated. Fluids are administered accordingly and the patient's response is monitored constantly. A concerted effort is made to minimize the patient's psychological and physiological stress. Attention is only directed to the actual burns when other aspects of care have been taken care of.

592. Keogh, Julian. "Management of Mass Burn Casualties in a Hospital with a Burn Unit." <u>Medical Journal of Australia</u> 1 (5 April 1980): 303-5.

   All hospital personnel, not only the burn unit personnel, must be prepared to cope with a mass burn disaster that would result in a sudden, unexpected, and large influx of patients. Good communication and transport systems would enable the transfer of patients to specialized units.

Literature

593. Krasnoff, Sidney O. "Statement on Criteria, Standards, and Data Requirements for the Appropriateness Review of Burn Care. Presented to Plan Development Committee of the Health Systems Agency of Southeastern Pennsylvania, June 23, 1980." Pennsylvania Medicine 76 (August 1980): 325.

594. McKinley, Joe C., et al. "Call for Help: An Algorithm for Burn Assessment, Triage and Acute Care." JACEP 5 (January 1976): 13-16.

   Because the Medical College of Georgia Burn Treatment Center frequently received patients with extensive burns who had been badly managed locally, an algorithm was devised to provide health care for professionals with a logical method for assessment, triage, and obtaining help. Limited experience suggests that the algorithm does, in fact, accomplish these ends but that continued evaluation of the efficacy is necessary. (Publication's Abstract)

595. Neal, Marie. "Thermal Injury Units in Rural Settings." Lamp 35 (December 1978-January 1979): 12-13.

   This paper considers the operation of centrally located thermal injury units in rural regions. Being located in base hospitals which serve an extended geographical area and provide specialist medical and nursing care to a number of smaller hospitals, there are problems in transport and communication. These are discussed and a structure for managing referrals is proposed. Problems encountered in rural areas are not merely small-scale versions of those found in urban hospitals; rather they are unique to their environmental setting.

596. Praise, Israel, et al. "The Planning and Organization of a Regionalized Burn Care System." Medical Care 18 (February 1980): 202-10.

   The National Burn Information Exchange's (NBIE) aims and function are described. The data compiled, organized, and analyzed at this institution are a major and valuable information resource for establishing criteria and policy guidelines for planning and implementing burn care services.

597. A Systems Approach to the Care of the Burn Victim. Grand Rapids, Mich.: EMS Patient Care Systems Planning and Implementation Symposia, November 11-13, 1975. Washington, D.C.: Department of Health, Education and Welfare, 1975. 36 p.

   It is the purpose of this collected paper on burn care to crystallize the medical-clinical concepts of a regionalized system of care for the critical burn patient by defining issues, current experience, and national perceptions for development of a sound response, care, and rehabilitation system for each patient category. This paper has been developed for discussion, exchange, and establishment of a beginning point for a national guidance program with subsequent modifications for local and regional program development.

Literature

598. Young, Steven R., and Thilliander, Brian D. "Patients, Staff are Focal Point of New Burn Unit." Hospitals 54 (16 February 1980): 93-99.

> The operation of the burn unit at Norfolk, Virginia, General Hospital is described. Some criteria for a good burn unit are posited: physical spaces and mechanical system must be designed to reduce infection, promote patient comfort, and improve staff efficiency and morale.

599. Wagner, Mary M. "Emergency Care of the Burned Patient." American Journal of Nursing 77 (November 1977): 1788-91.

> The focus of this article is that the burn victim must receive immediate care in the emergency department first, and there the patient has to be prepared for transfer to a burn center where definitive care will be initiated.

Spinal Cord Injury

Although a relatively uncommon injury, the permanent morbidity, long-term hospitalization, emotional impact, and extensive cost of care make this condition one of the most important EMS target patient categories. Experience indicates that systems of care for the spinal cord injured has brought substantial improvement in the process of care, its outcome, and in reduced cost.

600. Berger, Thomas S. "Acute Central Nervous System Emergencies." Ohio State Medical Journal 75 (June 1979): 345-46.

> This article deals with the imperative need for the development of regional centers for the care of critical neurologic patients. Reference sources are cited to justify the efficacy of such a system.

601. "A Comprehensive Plan for Spinal Cord Injury Services in Pennsylvania." Pennsylvania Medicine 81 (May 1978): 28-54.

> Spinal cord injury services in Pennsylvania are explained. Recommendations are: (1) that the Spinal Cord Injury Committee be reestablished under the secretary of health; (2) that the sum of two million dollars be allocated by legislation for implementing this proposal; (3) that the committee use these funds to (a) acquire an adequate full-time staff, (b) provide transportation, (c) provide for educational and developmental seed money; (4) that the committee be enabled to certify and approve spinal cord injury centers; (5) that the committee establish a mechanism for monitoring patient care, education, and research; and (6) that legislation be developed to make available facilities for handicapped individuals at educational institutions consistent with nondiscriminatory provision of section 504 of the Rehabilitation Act of 1973.

Literature

602. Hacen, H.J. "Idealized Care of the Acutely Injured Spinal Cord in Switzerland." Journal of Trauma 17 (December 1977): 931-36.

    The operation of the National Spinal Injuries Centre, Geneva University Hospital, Geneva, Switzerland, is described. Since the introduction of a helicopter rescue system in 1968, mortality rate dropped from 32.5 percent in 1966 to 6.8 percent in 1976.

603. Meyer, Paul R., Jr., and Raffensperger, John C. "Special Centers for the Care of the Injured." Journal of Trauma 13 (April 1973): 308-14.

    This article describes the historical background and actual operation of Chicago's Midwest Regional Spinal Injury Care System (MRSICS) and the Regional Pediatric Trauma Center in conjunction with the Illinois statewide trauma care system.

604. Schwentker, Edwards P., et al. "Coordinated Management of Spinal Cord Injuries." Pennsylvania Medicine 83 (September 1980): 39-41.

    The development and state of the art of spinal cord injured patients treatment are presented.

605. Wiseley, Sally F. "Clinical Management of Spinal Cord Injury: Experience in a Smaller State Rehabilitation Unit." Bulletin of the New York Academy of Medicine 55 (October 1979): 822-28.

    The concept that a spinal cord injury victim is best managed in a specialized unit with specialized staff, is forwarded. The author presents her experience at the Helen Hayes Hospital, Spinal Cord Unit, West Haverstraw, New York.

Poisoning

Poisoning occurs as a result of exposure to a very large number of toxic substances. The majority of toxic exposures can be handled over the phone by trained professionals within the Regional Poison Information and Control Center who give instructions to the public for patient management according to antidotal procedures. This consumer access system must include return telephone calls to insure effectiveness and patient safety as well as providing a link to inhospital providers.

606. "Emergency Medical Services Participation in Poison Control." National Clearinghouse Poison Control Center Bulletin 24 (June 1980): 5-6.

    This is a news release about the EMSS Act of 1979 and the operation of regional poison information and control centers.

607. Greensher, Joseph, and Mofeson, Howard C. "Emergency Room Care of the Poisoned Child." Issues in Comprehensive Pediatric Nursing 4 (June 1980): 1-21.

Literature

The incidence of child poisoning increases every year. Some can be considered accidental, others suicide attempts. This article describes how an emergency department has to be ready to deal with this kind of emergency.

608. Micik, Sylvia. "Emergency Medical Services and Poison Control." Clinical Toxicology 12 (March 1978): 309-17.

    The author presents her view on the system approach to Emergency Medical Services System. Only this system approach of patient care, as described in the EMSS Act of 1973 (PL 93-154), can decrease death and disability from medical emergencies. Poison care is but one part of the large chain.

609. _____. System Response to the Poisoned Patient. Grand Rapids, Mich.: EMS Patient Care System Planning and Implementation Symposia, November 11-13, 1975. 76 p.

    Each year in the United States an estimated five million poisonings occur, a number that is steadily increasing. Poisonings are the fourth most frequent cause of accidental death with only motor vehicle accidents, drownings, and burns more frequent. They result in over five thousand deaths per year, and a significant morbidity and disability at great cost to the nation. A total of 90 percent of the total reported cases involve children, making poisoning the most common pediatric medical emergency; the remaining 10 percent represent mostly suicide attempts, industrial poisonings, and drug abuse. These poisonings place a very large demand on our emergency medical resources, being responsible for 10 percent of all emergency room visits, and 5 to 10 percent of medical admissions.

610. Moriatry, Richard W. "Regionalization: The Pittsburgh Experience." Clinical Toxicology 12 (March 1978): 271-76.

    This is an account of the work of the Pittsburgh Poison Center and National Poison Center Network. The resource system provides analyzed data that help to deliver a more efficient service in poison and drug treatment and prevention.

611. Scherz, Robert G., and Robertson, William O. "The History of Poison Control Centers in the United States." Clinical Toxicology 12 (March 1978): 291-96.

    Poisoning is one main cause of infant and young child accidental death. Prevention and public education are two ways of reducing this type of injury. This article describes the history and the function of poison centers in the United States.

612. Temple, Anthony R., and Veltri, Joseph C. "One Year's Experience in a Regional Poison Control Center: The Intermountain Regional Poison Control Center." Clinical Toxicology 12 (March 1978): 277-89.

Literature

> The Intermountain Regional Poison Control Center, established in 1971, is a regional system that serves Utah, but also provides some cooperative services to neighboring states.

Acute Cardiac Care

Acute cardiac emergency is one of the most prevalent conditions seen within the EMS system. The EMS provides early intervention and cardiopulmonary resuscitation (CPR) at the scene. Basic life support procedures should be initiated as quickly as possible in the prehospital phase with further rapid integration to the emergency department and coronary care unit. Successful resuscitation of arrest victims requires rapid measures. American Heart Association criteria should be utilized when cardiac care designation of facilities and transportation units is done.

613. Lambrew, Costas T., et al. Critical Care Seminar Prospectus Emergency Cardiac Care. Grand Rapids, Mich.: EMS Patient Care Systems Planning and Implementation Symposia, November 11-13, 1975.

> The death rate from ischemic heart disease in the United States is 235.9 deaths per 100,000 population, nearly two times that of deaths from cancer, seven times the deaths from trauma. Development of the hospital coronary care unit has resulted in a decrease in hospital mortality from acute myocardial infarction (AMI) by 30 to 50 percent through early recognition and aggressive therapy of arrhythmias and consequent prevention of cardiac arrest. However, since 50 to 60 percent of deaths from coronary disease occur outside of the hospital, it is not surprising that the hospital coronary care unit has not substantially decreased community mortality from acute coronary events. Pantridge, in Belfast, pioneered the extension of the coronary care unit to the prehospital phase and demonstrated a reduction in prehospital mortality from acute myocardial infarction through stabilization of the patient at the scene of the incident and en route to hospital.

614. Wheeler, E. Todd. "Establishing Sizes for I.C.U., C.C.U., Outpatient and Emergency Units." Hospital Topics 51 (October 1973): 35-39.

> This paper presents a method of establishing the proper sizes of four hospital departments--intensive care unit, coronary care unit, ambulatory patient department, and emergency department. It is a hypothetical study for a 375-bed acute general hospital, located in a city of one million inhabitants, with fifteen other hospitals, including a county-city hospital and three medical school hospitals.

High Risk Infant

The EMS system, in improving the transportation and care of the high-risk infant, should be planned within the framework of the overall state perinatal plan. The plan developed should make provision for definition of health ser-

Literature

vice regions as well as provide guidelines for regional planning activities.

615. Callon, Helen F. "Regionalizing Perinatal Care in Wisconsin." Nursing Clinics of North America 10 (June 1975): 263-74.

> Faced with the high percentage of neonatal deaths (as recently as 1967, world statistics ranked the United States nineteenth), Wisconsin medical organizations decided to systematize and regionalize their facilities to decrease perinatal deaths.

616. Chance, Graham W., et al. "Neonatal Transport: A Controlled Study of Skilled Assistance." Journal of Pediatrics 93 (October 1978): 662-66.

> A controlled study of infants being transported to the Neonatal Intensive Care Unit, Hospital for Sick Children, Toronto, illustrated that sick neonates need skilled care en route to the hospital. Ambulances were not modified but specialized equipment was utilized.

617. Comprehensive Health Planning Agency of Southern Wisconsin. Guidelines for Neo-Natal Intensive Care Units. Milwaukee: May 1971. 13 p. (NTIS HRP-0003952)

> Optimum criteria for establishment of neonatal intensive care units in southeastern Wisconsin are presented. The following factors are considered: staffing (registered and licensed practical nurses and physicians); physical facility requirements; minimum desirable case load; relationship of the neonatal intensive care unit to other hospital programs and to other hospitals; physician and allied health personnel training; and patient follow-up. An outline for use in identifying high-risk pregnancies is included.

618. Hackel, Alvin. "A Medical Transport System for the Neonate." Anesthesiology 43 (August 1975): 258-67.

> This paper describes the Stanford Newborn Intensive Care Nurseries. This service has been utilized as a regional facility for more than two decades. It covers an area with a radius of 150 to 250 miles, fifty-six hospitals and about forty-eight hundred deliveries a year.

619. Herrera, Alfredo J., et al. "Newborn Land Transport: The St. Agnes Hospital Experience." Maryland State Medical Journal 29 (September 1980): 58-59.

> One year's progress of the St. Agnes Hospital, Baltimore, newborn land transportation system is described.

620. Horobo, Roberta Gatjen. Emergency Care of the Critically Ill Newborn Infant. Palo Alto, Calif.: Stanford University, Department of Anesthesia, 1974. 222 p. (NTIS HRP-0004411)

Literature

A twenty-month project aimed at improving emergency care for critically ill newborn infants in a fifteen-county area of northern California is reported by the Stanford University Medical Center community coordinator. The objectives of the project were: to improve recognition and emergency management of catastrophic illness in newborns in the secondary care setting; to design and implement a continuing education program in emergency medical care of critically ill newborns for the professional team in the secondary care setting; to develop a coordinated communication system between secondary and tertiary care centers; to develop an effective interim transport module to allow intensive care in a controlled environment en route to the tertiary care center; to study the existing emergency transportation system and develop a model system for transport of critically ill newborns needing emergency care; and to develop formalized linkages for emergency services to newborns and children of other age groups with the community hospitals of the region.

621. Mazzi, Eduardo, and Gutberlet, Ronald. "The Maryland State Intensive Care Neonatal Program (MSICNP): Description and One-Year Evaluation." Maryland State Medical Journal 26 (November 1977): 61-65.

This article is an evaluation of the Maryland State Intensive Care Neonatal Program.

622. Mazzi, Eduardo, et al. "The Maryland State Intensive Care Neonatal Program (MSICNP). Part 2: Role of the Maryland State Police Aviation Division." Maryland State Medical Journal 26 (December 1977): 48-50.

During twelve months, 341 infants were transferred to Baltimore neonatal centers from different hospitals throughout Maryland and neighboring states as well; 76 percent of the infants were transferred by helicopter and almost 60 percent were without physician accompaniment. The basic transport team consists of a well-trained pilot and a paramedic with physician assistance in selected cases.

623. _____. "The Maryland State Intensive Care Neonatal Program (MSICNP). Part 3: The Role of the Nursing Department." Maryland State Medical Journal 27 (January 1978): 75-77.

The role of the nursing department in the Maryland State Intensive Care Neonatal Program is described.

624. Rossi, E.A. "Emergency Transport Service for Sick Newborn." Schweizerische Medizinsche Wochenschrift 105 (1975): 1210-15.

An emergency transportation service for sick newborns in the region of Berne, Switzerland, is described. It is manned by a specialized team consisting of pediatric resident and a pediatric intensive care nurse. Of the 135 newborns transported in 1974, 8 were by helicopter and the rest by ambulance.

Literature

625. Staub, Gerald F., et al. "The High Risk Perinatal (Neonatal) Patient." Grand Rapids, Michigan, EMS Patient Care Systems Design and Implementation Symposia, November 11-13, 1975. 110 p. (Publication is forthcoming).

> Although the systems approach is unique for the high-risk neonatal patient because it must include a perinatal (mother-fetus-newborn) orientation, the organization and practical application of that approach does permit inclusion of the appropriate components of an Emergency Medical Service System. Organization of the system should begin ideally and practically with a state-wide plan for perinatal health which is integrated with the EMS plan for the entire state. The development of the state-wide plan should be the responsibility of the state department of public health, the state comprehensive planning agency, and an appropriate perinatal planning group having a broad cross-sectional professional geographic representation.

626. Zachman, Richard D., and Graven, Stanley N. "A Neonatal Intensive Care Unit." American Journal of Diseases of Children 128 (August 1974): 165-70.

> The authors report on the first four years' experience of the Neonatal Intensive Care Unit in Madison, Wisconsin. This facility is located in a community hospital and includes a normal newborn nursery, an observation unit, and an intensive care unit.

Behavioral Emergencies

The system must coordinate a comprehensive range of medical and social services in cooperation with existing institutions and agencies for those individuals experiencing psychosocial trauma.

The system should plan for care of alcoholism, drug abuse, suicide, rape, and other behavioral emergencies.

627. Danto, Bruce L. "MD Handling Psychiatric Emergencies Must Give Specific, Caring Treatment." Michigan Medicine 78 (February 1979): 64.

> A physician attending a psychiatric emergency must be very careful in order to find out if the patient requires specific treatment which is not available in the average emergency department.

628. Frazier, William H., and Moynihan, Barbara. "The Emergency Service Based Rape Counseling Team." Connecticut Medicine 42 (February 1978): 91-94.

> The Rape Counseling Team at the Yale-New Haven Hospital was developed in order to coordinate the diverse services required in providing effective care to victims of sexual assault. In two and one-half years, utilization of the team has increased by 600 percent.

Literature

629. Ghodse, A. Hamid. "Recommendations by Accident and Emergency Staff About Drug-Overdose Patients." Social Science and Medicine 13A (March 1979): 169-73.

> In a survey, doctors and nurses employed by London Accident and Emergency Departments recommended methods for dealing with drug overdose cases. The majority concurred that the patients should be evaluated and advised by a resident psychiatrist. Sum of 66 percent thought a security guard should be present in the emergency department; 79 percent believed that special emergency facilities should be established to handle drug-related cases; and 60 percent backed a voluntary ban on barbituate prescriptions.

630. Huddleston, William C. "System Response to Behavioral Emergencies." Grand Rapids, Michigan, EMS Patient Care Systems Design and Implementation Symposia, November 11-13, 1975. 111 p. (Publication forthcoming).

> When one contemplates the integration of the "behavioral emergency patient" into the overall structure of emergency medical services, he or she is immediately confronted with the problem of establishing adequate definitions. Much debate has centered around the question of whether the traditional phrase "psychiatric emergency" should be used to encompass all types of mental and emotional crises including, but not limited to, acute alcoholism, drug overdose, child neglect, family conflict, aggressive problem behavior, depressive-suicidal behavior, and hysterical behavior of bystanders at the scene of the emergency. Many strong arguments have been advanced asserting that the term "psychiatric" is too restrictive for such a broad category of emergency services. It has been suggested that more appropriate categorization might be "mental health emergencies," "severe emotional crisis," or even "ADAMHA" (Alcohol, Drug Abuse, and Mental Health Administration) related emergencies.

631. Josephson, Gordon W. "The Male Rape Victim: Evaluation and Treatment." JACEP 8 (January 1979): 13-15.

> The medical literature offers little guidance in the evaluation of male victims of sexual assault. The statutes are a confusing patchwork of conflicting and sexually biased laws. The evaluation and treatment of the sexually abused male victim is similar to his female counterpart. Physicians and emergency department staff must be knowledgeable regarding their responsibilities to these patients, and concerned with the medical, legal, and psychological ramifications of sexual assault.

632. Southeast Arkansas Economic Development District. Southeast Arkansas District Plan for the Prevention, Treatment, and Control of Alcohol Abuse and Alcoholism. Pine Bluff, Ark.: Areawide Health Planning Program, January 1975. 92 p. (NTIS HRP-0004551)

A plan for the prevention and treatment of alcoholism in ten southeastern Arkansas counties is presented. The planning area contains the second most populated county in the state as well as several of the most sparsely populated counties. Area residents tend to be far below average in income and education. Blacks comprise 35.98 percent of the population. In 1972 the northern catchment area had 2.56 admissions to alcoholic treatment sites per 1,000 population, while the southern catchment area had 0.63 admissions per 1,000. State average was 1.03 admissions per 1,000.

633. Zimberg, Sheldon. "Alcoholism: Prevalence in General Hospital Emergency Room and Walk-in-Clinic." New York State Journal of Medicine 79 (September 1979): 1533-36.

A study revealed an alcoholism prevalence rate of 28 percent among walk-in clinic patients and 31 and 38 percent among emergency room patients at the Hospital for Joint Diseases and Medical Center, New York. Because physicians staffing the walk-in clinic and emergency room generally demonstrate a pessimistic attitude about alcoholism treatment, few of the patients are referred. The study recommends the addition of alcoholism counselors to these services.

Public Safety Agencies

The system must involve in its function all public safety agencies, police, fire fighters, lifeguards, park rangers, and other appropriate public safety personnel. All these services have to be adequately coordinated to render the best utilization of personnel, facilities, and equipment. Plans have to be set up to develop cooperative operating procedures among services on a day-to-day basis, as well as during major disasters.

634. Page, James O. Emergency Medical Services for Fire Departments. Boston: National Fire Protection Association, 1975. 300 p.

This important book marks a new era in fire department operations. In very specific detail, it describes how fire departments are expanding their efforts into emergency medical services, despite the obstacles of tradition and the normal reluctance of communities to divert tax revenues into a new field of public service. Yet, as the author contends, perhaps no other municipal organization than the fire department is better prepared for Emergency Medical Services, because few groups have as many direct, constant encounters with the public. In more than one hundred years of operation, the U.S. Fire Service has been closely identified with the rescue and care of the victims of tragic fires and other disasters. It seems natural for the members of fire departments to respond to the challenge of rendering emergency care to injured and stricken victims. (Author's Introduction)

635. _____. "EMS and the Fire Service." Fire Command 41 (August 1974): 60-70.

Literature

Many firemen consider EMS as a threat to their traditional status. In the light of PL 93-154, the Emergency Medical Services Act of 1973, Chief Page discusses the role of the fire service in emergency medical services.

Consumer Participation

The system has to ensure that people residing in the area, with no professional training or experience, participate in the policymaking of the system. Consumers also must have access to policymakers to register complaints and constructive criticism in regard to the planning, operation, and implementation of the system.

636. "Emergency Medical Council Ready to Act in Central Indiana." Journal of the Indiana State Medical Association 71 (September 1978): 814.

> The Central Indiana Emergency Medical Services Council plan for operation is described. This council serves an eight-county area.

637. Heidt, Robert S. "Organization of Emergency Medical Services Councils." Ohio State Medical Journal 70 (June 1974): 352-56.

> The article relates in general terms the reasons and needs to organize an EMS council. The main components are also detailed.

638. Novack, Margit. Improving Emergency Services Through Community Involvement. Philadelphia: Center for the Study of Emergency Health Services, May 1974. 21 p.

> Increasingly, emergency departments have become the focus of patient dissatisfaction with institutional health services, as well as professional distress at the inappropriate utilization of the emergency facility for nonurgent cases. The Graduate Hospital of the University of Pennsylvania established an Emergency Service Community Advisory Board (GESCAB) to address both of these problems. The goal of the community advisory board is to improve emergency services by creating a better relationship between the community and the EMS staff through a reciprocal educational process. Study covers 8 November 1973 to 8 April 1974.

639. Nutt, Paul Charles. "Some Considerations in Selecting Interactive and Analytical Decision Approaches for EMS Councils." Medical Care 17 (February 1979): 152-67.

> The application of analytical and interactive models to decisions, in EMS councils, with various levels of uncertainty is described. The results of applying interactive and analytical decision models under varying levels of uncertainty are discussed. (Abbreviated Author's Abstract)

Literature

640. Paetow, Paul F. "Community Emergency Care Advisory Councils: How They Work, What They Accomplish." Bulletin American College of Surgeons 55 (January 1970): 19-21, 25.

   Many EMS councils were formed following the motto: "Get the community involved." Many of these organizations are statewide in composition, others are purely local. This report assesses some of the more important features of five such councils.

641. Rumage, William T. "Your Community Emergency Medical Services Council." Archives Environmental Health 21 (August 1970): 211-13.

   The author posits the following council responsibilities: (1) organize community response; (2) organize medical response to evaluate and treat patients in disaster; (3) community-wide communication facilities; (4) program to train; and, (5) supplies and equipment.

642. Schroeder, Oliver G., Jr. "Health Consumers and Medical Practitioners: Is Conflict Inevitable?" Postgraduate Medicine 53 (April 1973): 203-5.

   Consumers are demanding--and getting--a stronger voice in decisions affecting health care delivery. Greater consumer participation and education should alleviate conflicts with medical practitioners arising from high medical costs, complexity of the health care system, and consumer militancy.

643. Sparacino, Sharon H. "Involving the Public in EMS." JEN 1 (July-August 1975): 28-30.

   The article describes the Public Safety Officers Foundation's massive effort to instruct the lay public in cardiopulmonary resuscitation.

644. Stratmann, William C., and Ullman, Ralph. "A Study of Consumer Attitudes about Health Care: The Role of the Emergency Room." Medical Care 13 (December 1975): 1033-41.

   The authors report in this article on public opinion about the role of the emergency department; the perceived urgency of the problems that people bring to the emergency department; the accessibility of medical care; and factors that prompt the utilization of the emergency department rather than other types of medical facilities.

F. ACCESSIBILITY TO CARE

The system must provide, without prior inquiry as to ability to pay, necessary emergency medical services to all patients requiring such services. The access must be assured for ambulance services, initial general hospital care, secondary transport to critical care units, and rehabilitation centers.

Literature

645. Acton, Jan Paul. <u>Demand for Health Care Among the Urban Poor with Special Emphasis on the Role of Time.</u> New York: Prepared for the U.S. Office of Economic Opportunity and the New York City Health Services Administration by Rand Institution, April 1973. 52 p. (R-1151-E/NYC)

> This study examines the demand for medical services by type of provider with particular emphasis on the role of time as a determining factor. The demand for health and medical services has attracted considerable interest in recent years because of the dramatic increase in health expenditures and because of substantial cost inflation in that sector.

646. American Hospital Association. <u>A Patient's Bill of Rights.</u> Chicago: 1973. 6 p.

> This document consists of twelve articles delineating what the AHA considers to be the rights of all patients.

G. COORDINATED PATIENT RECORD KEEPING

A standardized patient record keeping meeting appropriate standards must be implemented in each emergency medical services system. The record should include data of the patient from initial entry into the system through his/her discharge, that is: prehospital, hospital, and critical care unit within the system.

647. Abrams, Jerome, and Davis, John H. "Advantages of the Problem-Oriented Medical Record in the Care of the Severely Injured Patient." <u>Journal of Trauma</u> 14 (May 1974): 361-69.

> The POMR, Problem-Oriented Medical Record, has resulted in significant improvement in the overall care of traumatized patients. This article delineates the advantages of POMR in the study of diagnosis management.

648. Alber, Philip R. "The Problem-Oriented Record: It's Not for Me." <u>Medical Economics</u> 52 (6 January 1975): 69-73.

> The author catalogues and discusses, from his point of view, the disadvantages of the problem-oriented medical record (POMR).

649. Ayers, W.R., et al. "Mobilizing the Emergency Room Record: A Case Study in the Capture of Technology Developed Elsewhere for Use in Health Care Delivery." <u>Computer Biological Medicine</u> 3 (1973): 153-63.

> The Georgetown University Pediatric Pulmonary Program developed an automated Emergency Department patient record. The on-line, commercially available, time-shared system was used by four hospitals. No new technology was required for the system. Rather, existing technical capability was transferred for use in a medical setting. A revised version

Literature

of the system is now being experimented within private physician offices, county medical clinics, and the university pediatric center.

650. Birch, H. <u>Guidelines for Patient Record-Keeping Systems for Emergency Medical Service.</u> 2 vols. Silver Spring, Md.: Macro Systems, 1974. (PB-243 781)

   The main aspects covered are the need for record keeping standards, the state of the art with respect to EMS patient record keeping systems, a description of the management information needs of local EMS program managers, and the national program. A minimum dataset is also included.

651. Boyd, David R. "Trauma Registry: New Computer Method for Multifactorial Evaluation of a Major Health Problem." <u>Journal of the American Medical Association</u> 223 (22 January 1973): 422-28.

   This article is an expansion of the above-cited entry.

652. _____, et al. "Computerized Trauma Registry: A New Method for Categorizing Physical Injuries." <u>Aerospace Medicine</u> 42 (1971): 607-15.

   A central trauma registry was developed at the trauma unit of the Cook County Hospital and Research Resources Laboratory of the University of Illinois, using an IBM 360/44 computer and a generalized information retrieval system. The registry employs a card-oriented data collection procedure, but will utilize direct entry from remote video terminals. Information is collected on epidemiologic factors and extent of anatomical damage, as well as operative treatment employed and specific complications encountered. The International Classification of Disease (adopted 1969) categories are integrated into the registry, but a new tabulation system is being utilized as the prime patient indexing method.

653. Cayten, C. Gene, and Evans, William. "Severity Indices and Their Implications for Emergency Medical Services Research and Evaluation." <u>Journal of Trauma</u> 19 (February 1979): 98-102.

   The rationale for the development of severity indexes and the role such indexes can play in various research and evaluation situations is explored.

654. Cole, Linda, et al. "Prehospital Cardiac Care: Illusion of Concensus." JACEP 6 (December 1977): 552-55.

   To judge standard practice for managing arrhythmias, what an EMT should be able to do in the field, drugs of choice, the success of EMT training, and the quality of EMT performance, clinical algorithms were developed. Branching logic, forcing yes-no decisions and delineating actions for all contingencies helped formalize and systematize EMT management of urgent and emergency cases. The algorithm set

Literature

was sent to nineteen consultants for review of content, sequence, drug dosage, and drug usage. The results indicated lack of consensus on appropriate prehospital cardiac care, but indicated the approval of the algorithm approach.

655. Eisenberg, Mickey S., et al. "Out-of-Hospital Cardiac Arrest: A Review of Major Studies and a Proposed Uniform Reporting System." American Journal of Public Health 70 (March 1980): 236-40.

> A review of the literature from 1970 to 1979 reveals that there has been no uniform procedure for reporting outcomes from out-of-hospital cardiac arrest treated by paramedic programs. This paper recommends and describes a simplified, standard reporting format.

656. George, James E. "The ED Record: Friend or Foe?" JACEP 5 (July 1976): 535-40.

> Emergency department record requirements are more stringent today than a few years ago. Federally supported programs mandate complete ED record keeping. Accrediting organizations, such as the Joint Commission on Accreditation of Hospitals, established one of the most comprehensive ED record keeping procedures. The author attempts to familiarize the emergency physician with the medicolegal implications of the ED record.

657. Gibson, Geoffrey. "Indices of Severity of Emergency Medical Evaluative Studies: Reliability, Validity, and Data Requirements." Presented at the Annual Meeting of the American College of Emergency Physicians, New Orleans, October 1976. 53 p.

> Three sets of methodologic requirements, reliability, validity, and data requirements, are suggested and used to evaluate the methodologic adequacy of seventeen commonly used severity indexes. In general, the indexes were found to depend on clinical subjective judgments, to lack clear or objective definitions, to offer little evidence that they could be used reliably. While all correlated with mortality, few had a documented ability to predict morbidity. Most indexes had not been validated prospectively and retrospectively nor been tested in different settings. Thus, they may be substantially contaminated by the idiosyncratic patient mix in the facility and series used for scale development, and not generalizable as a severity measure to other populations. Only five of the seventeen indexes met even minimal methodologic criteria used.

658. Gustafson, David H., and Holloway, Donald C. "A Decision Theory Approach to Measuring Severity in Illness." Health Services Research 10 (Spring 1975): 97-106.

> The purpose of this study was to evaluate the applicability of a multiattribute utility model for measuring the severity of a patient's illness. A single medical problem, an analysis of the costs and benefits of different burn care systems, was used to test the model.

Literature

659. Herrmann, Nira, et al. "Interobserver and Intraobserver Reliability in the Collection of Emergency Medical Services Data." Health Services Research 15 (Summer 1980): 127-43.

> This paper reports on a study of patient data abstracted from emergency department records by nurses trained by project personnel. The results demonstrate that even well-trained, motivated abstractors exhibit considerable differences in the accuracy with which they abstract the variables. This paper makes several suggestions for improving the quality of abstracted data: better hospital record retrieval procedures, monitoring of data collection methods, cooperation of all medical personnel providing the raw data, and careful selection of variables.

660. Kaufman, Theodore, et al. "Auditing Care with a Problem-Oriented Record System." JACEP 4 (September-October 1975): 416-18.

> This is a study at Beth Israel Medical Center to evaluate emergency department care. Findings show that auditors could review problem-oriented records in less time and in greater numbers than traditional medical records.

661. Krischer, Jeffrey P. "Indexes of Severity: Conceptual Development." Health Services Research 14 (Spring 1979): 56-67.

> This paper discusses severity index development as it relates to conceptual issues in index definition, analytical issues in index formulation, and validation issues in index application.

662. O'Neill, Brian, et al. "Indexes of Severity: Underlying Concepts--A Reply." Health Services Research 14 (Spring 1979): 68-76.

> A recent article on the ideas underlying indexes of severity that have been proposed for health services research claimed to point out weaknesses in each. Careful scrutiny shows that the criticisms are generally unfounded, and that the claim that the indexes "violate some of the principles implied by their formulation" is erroneous. Most of the objections are an apparent result of fundamental confusion about the use of such indexes.

663. "The Problem-Oriented Record: Try It and You'll Like It." Medical Economics, 6 January 1975, pp. 74-78.

> This article outlines the advantages of the problem-oriented medical record (POMR).

664. Rosati, Robert A., et al. "A New Information System for Medical Practice." Archives Internal Medicine 135 (August 1975): 1017-24.

> A databank of three thousand patients with suspected and documented ischemic heart disease was used to expand patient care ability. This experience was documented, stored, and retrieved so that it can be used in patient management. Data

Literature

acquisition is integrated with patient care by means of forms that are part of the patient record. All data are stored in a computer information system that allows the physician to recall the experience of patients like his/her new patient.

665. Roussi, C.C., and Maxwell, David M. "An Improved Record System for the Emergency Department." JACEP 4 (September-October 1975): 419-25.

    A two-component system designed to circumvent many of the problems inherent in emergency department record keeping is described. First, a packet of multiple forms interleaved with carbon paper allows copies of all relevant data to be produced for distribution, including to the follow-up physician, simultaneously. Second, physicians use a hand-held portable dictating machine with mini-cassettes to dictate each patient's history on a separate cassette. The record is typed from the cassette by a transcription typist based in the emergency department. Thus, a typewritten record of the patient's visit, including prescription for medications, is produced before the patient leaves the department. (Author's Abstract)

666. Schwartz, George R. "The Emergency Department Record." JACEP 3 (November-December 1974): 385-87.

    Fifty emergency department records were evaluated against certain criteria developed within the Medical College of Pennsylvania. A model record system was developed to meet actual needs of patients and emergency department administration.

667. Steele, Richard, et al. Development of a Minimum Data Set for Emergency Medical Services Patient Recordkeeping. Silver Spring, Md.: Macro Systems, July 1974. 72 p. (NTIS PB-243-822)

    This final report is a result of a federal initiative to upgrade EMSSs in the United States, in particular the section of the law that requires standardized patient record keeping systems. HSA determined that the requirements of the law could be met by instructing each EMSS grantee to collect a specified and limited list of data items. This report discusses the approach and methodology of a minimum EMS data set.

668. U.S. Department of Health, Education and Welfare. Division of Emergency Medical Services. EMS Handbook for Patient Recordkeeping and List of Minimum Data. West Hyattsville, Md.: August 1977. 42 p. (HSA 77-2034)

    The list of minimum data contains those elements which are applicable to a decision-making process within an EMS system. They are appropriate for such activities as planning, control, and evaluation. This data set can be adjusted according to local needs.

Literature

669. Valbona, Carlos, and Evans, Lynn. <u>Emergency Care Quality: Usefulness of Patient Profiles.</u> Houston: Baylor College of Medicine, December 1976. 51 p. (NTIS PB-272 369)

   The purpose of this project was to demonstrate improvement in the quality of emergency medical care, primarily in terms of appropriateness, completeness, and cost-benefit, by providing emergency physicians at a large metropolitan hospital with a concise summary of the patient's previous medical record (a Health-Illness Profile [H-IP]). The results of this study demonstrated no impact of the H-IP on the classification of case abstracts before and after having access to H-IP data.

670. Wenzel, V., et al. "Evaluating the Pre-Hospital Phase of the Emergency Medical System." <u>Virginia Medical</u> 106 (November 1979): 858-59.

   This paper reviews the development and progress of a standardized ambulance report form, in Virginia Planning District 10, and addresses its role in evaluating the prehospital phase of the EMS system.

H. PUBLIC INFORMATION AND EDUCATION

Programs of public education and information in the system's service area must be developed so the public will know about the system, how to access it, and how to use it.

Programs also have to be developed that will stress the general information regarding appropriate methods of medical self-help and first aid and regarding the availability of first aid training programs in the area.

671. American Trauma Society. <u>Emergency Medical Services Public Information Manual.</u> Chicago: September 1978. 35 p.

   This manual was compiled as a working draft for the EMS Public Education and Information Symposium, September 11-13, 1978.

672. Arkansas Health Systems Foundation. <u>Consumer Information and Education Handbook for the Emergency Medical Services System.</u> Little Rock: 1973. 37 p. (NTIS HRP-0005723)

   This handbook is designed primarily for local use, but offers general information, examples, and suggestions for planning a consumers' information and education program. Topics covered include writing a news release, calling a press conference, and listing of public education materials. The second section describes in considerable detail the Basic Rural Outreach Model, which has proven effective in rural areas.

673. Campbell, Donald A., and Raming, Nancy D. <u>Public Education and Information for Emergency Medical Services Development. The Southeast Ohio Experience.</u> Columbus: Ohio State University, Department of Preventive Medicine, June 1976. 163 p. (NTIS PB-261 442)

Literature

The report is divided primarily into five sections. Section 1 is a brief summary of current trends in EMS development nationally and the relevance of public education and information to this undertaking. Section 2 includes a brief description of the SEOEMS demonstration project and a review of the program plan for public education and information. Section 3 is a review of the principle programs and activities of the SEOEMS educational effort. Section 4 deals with public information, community organization, and citizen participation; and Section 5 includes a summary and general recommendations. Several of the public education programs developed in the course of the project and selected educational resources which proved to be useful in carrying out the program are included in the appendixes.

674. "Emergency Information at Community's Doors." Hospitals 47 (1 July 1973): 28.

Spanish-speaking and Greek-speaking communities of northside Chicago now have an information source that will help them to the appropriate service in case of emergency. This information is contained in a trilingual brochure--English, Greek, and Spanish.

675. First, Joan M., et al. Data Profiles EMS Public Awareness and Utilization Patterns in Arkansas. Arkansas Health Statistics Center Technical Reports, no. 2. Little Rock: Arkansas Health Systems Foundation, January 1974. 10 p. (NTIS PB-250 794)

This is an Arkansas study of families' awareness of various aspects of the EMS system that serves them and of their knowledge about what to do in case of an emergency. Data was obtained through a state-wide household survey. Two-thirds of families surveyed have not discussed the possibility of a medical emergency. In 31 percent of the sample, word of mouth represented the main source of EMS information. The next group, 23 percent, used the telephone book. Knowledge of specific ambulance services was limited, but 84 percent named hospitals as the usual source of emergency care, with doctors' offices the next most frequently cited sources.

676. National EMS Information Clearinghouse. Emergency Medical Services Public Education Guidebook. Philadelphia: University of Pennsylvania, Center for the Study of Emergency Health Services, 1976. 62 p.

This guidebook, based on extensive review of the literature and existing programs, is intended to assist communities in designing and implementing a public education program, especially in urban areas. Chapters deal with: definition of public education, discussion of methods, planning principle, and finally, a step-by-step action plan. Appendixes include references and sources of information in both public education and EMS.

Literature

677. Superior California Comprehensive Health System. Emergency Medical Services Consumer Information and Education. <u>A Manual for Developing Community Programs.</u> Chico: 1974. 113 p.

   This manual was distributed to all county EMC committees in California in order to share some of the ideas and methods tested in Tehama County. Following a presentation of the conceptual framework and description of organizational methods, the manual focuses on an EMS Information Center (EMSIC) as the vehicle for public education. An extensive appendix includes: sources of information, household interview survey (Spanish and English), standards for CPR, and basic life support.

I. REVIEW AND EVALUATION

Periodic, comprehensive, and independent review and evaluation of the extent and quality of emergency health care services must be conducted in the system's service area.

678. Alvin, Susan L., et al. "Evaluation of Emergency Room Triage Performed by Nurses." <u>American Journal of Public Health</u> 65 (October 1975): 1963-68.

   This is an evaluation of the effectiveness of specially trained nurses in performing triage for incoming patients at the Bronx Municipal Hospital Center emergency department. The nurses received their training after one year of general experience in emergency nursing. The importance of properly trained triage personnel, ongoing monitoring of triage errors, and subsequent reeducation is stressed.

679. Anderson, Gail V., et al. "A Unique Approach to Evaluation of Emergency Care." JACEP 6 (June 1977): 254-58.

   A quality of care evaluation process was designed to serve as a framework for a research in quality assurance in emergency medical services. The assessment was done using procedures such as direct observation of patient, review and analysis of patient medical record, and patient follow-up interview for outcome. The research intended to show relationships between quality of care and patient outcome.

680. Andrews, Robert B., et al. <u>Methodologies for the Evaluation and Improvement of Emergency Medical Services Systems: Final Report.</u> Los Angeles: University of California, Graduate School of Management, Division of Research, July 1975. 568 p. (NTIS PB-244 462)

   This project demonstrated methodologies for the evaluation of existing and proposed systems for the delivery of emergency medical services. An appreciative overview is presented which analyzes emergency medical services in terms of a historical perspective; the evolving social, cultural, and technical environment in which they are embedded;

Literature

how they are viewed by the users, health professionals, and provider organizations; and the forces that tend to facilitate and to inhibit their change.

681. Arthur Young and Co. Evaluation Workbook for EMS. Washington, D.C.: 1976. Var. pag.

   This workbook is a set of guidelines to help managers of Emergency Medical Services Systems to perform evaluation in light of the thirteenth component of the EMSS Public Act of 1973.

682. Bachrach, Peter. Evaluation of the Effectiveness of Emergency Medical Services Councils in Wisconsin. Madison: Wisconsin Regional Medical Programs, April 1976. 117 p. (NTIS HRP-0011220)

   The effectiveness of eight area-wide emergency medical services councils in Wisconsin is assessed. The councils, organized under the aegis of comprehensive health planning agencies, were funded by the Wisconsin Regional Medical Program through the Wisconsin EMS program from July 1972 through June 1975. Composed of volunteers, staffed by an EMS coordinator, and charged with the responsibility of improving the delivery of emergency care, these councils approached their task differently. The method used to evaluate the EMS councils is described.

683. Blum, Marc S., and Stone, Linda S. Evaluation of Emergency Medical Services Systems Impact. Atlanta: Transaction Systems, 1975. 23 p. (NTIS PB-243 714)

   This project analyzed and evaluated the capabilities of existing regional EMS systems in their delivery of specific emergency medical care needs throughout the nation. The scope of the project included the gathering of pertinent data to aid in the evaluation and analysis of the need and the level of need of certain specialized health delivery systems within the EMS system and to determine whether or not these regional systems make a difference on mortality and morbidity statistics.

684. Boldt, Ronald, et al. Analysis of Ambulance Service Needs in Yuba-Sutter Counties. Superior: California Comprehensive Health Planning Association, December 1973. 21 p. (NTIS HRP-0004318)

   The economic feasibility of adding a third ambulance service in Sutter and Yuba Counties, California, as well as the impact such an addition would have on the quality of emergency medical care in the counties, are considered in this report. Existing emergency care resources in the area are assessed, including an inventory of ambulance vehicles and equipment. The proposed third service in the two counties is determined. Costs of the existing two services are estimated, and the cost of adding a third service is projected.

Literature

685. Bovier, F. "The Development and Application of a Management Tool for the Analysis of Hospital Emergency Room Functions." Master's thesis, Rensselaer Polytechnic Institute, Troy, New York, 1972. 204 p.

> This work describes the development and implementation of a management procedure for analyzing hospital emergency department functions. Some of the aspects evaluated are: patient case load, staff workload, ancillary services impact, and admission statistics.

686. Cayten, C. Gene, and Thomas, J. William. EMS Planning and Evaluation. Philadelphia: University of Pennsylvania, Center for the Study of Emergency Health Services, 1974. 27 p.

> Emergency medical care, in most of the country, is but an accumulation of uncoordinated services. Only recently the need for EMS planning has been acknowledged. The benefits of a planned EMS system are many; but those benefits also create problems. This paper illustrates the basic procedures for planning an EMS system and for performing ongoing evaluation. The following topics are addressed: the scope of EMS; the EMS planning process; program evaluation information and feedback; general EMS evaluation method; and information systems for EMS planning and evaluation.

687. Cayten, C. Gene, et al. "Assessing the Validity of EMS Data." JACEP 7 (November 1978): 390-96.

> Variation in the assessment of basic clinical data gathered by emergency medical technicians and emergency department nurses was studied. Prior to testing, precise definitions, categories, and procedures were developed and tolerance limits for the quantitative variables were created. Each participant evaluated four consecutive patients simultaneously with another evaluator setting the standard. The results indicate that the error rate is low to moderate for the different variables. For the quantitative variables, the error rate is over 20 percent and, when an error does occur, it is often very large. This indicates a need for ongoing emphasis on accurate measurement and, in cases where highly accurate data is essential, the use of multiple observers. (Author's Abstract)

688. Cole, Linda, et al. "Auditing the Quality of Care in Emergency Departments." JACEP 5 (January 1976): 32-35.

> The purpose of this project was to develop a methodology for evaluating the quality of care in emergency departments. An audit of retrospective emergent and urgent cases was developed and tested in the Philadelphia General Hospital's emergency department. From the twelve most common chief complaints, six were selected as representative, and a panel of experts developed explicit criteria which were checked against current medical literature for clinical soundness.

Literature

689. Computer Science Corp. <u>An Evaluation Methodology for Emergency Medical Services Systems.</u> Paramus, N.J.: June 1973. 205 p. (NTIS PB-221 605)

> The object of this program was to study various methods for developing EMS data on which governmental decision making might be based. After the study, one method was chosen and developed into a complete EMS assessment model. Work started with a baseline questionnaire developed under NATO. This was refined, expanded, and field tested in a number of states with the intention that, under NATO, it might become an international standard for EMS assessment. Appropriate effectiveness measures are described and a weighting system in which mathematical totals can be derived is suggested.

690. Daley, Edward V. "Economic Evaluation of Alternative Emergency Medical Services Systems in Columbia, Missouri." Ph.D. dissertation, Middle Tennessee State University, Murfreesboro, May 1974. 121 p.

> Criteria that can be used to evaluate an emergency medical service system were presented and the use of these criteria is demonstrated. The <u>Highway Safety Program Manual,</u> (Washington, D.C.: Government Printing Office, January 1969) and Supplement 1, (February 1971), developed in response to the National Highway Safety Act of 1966, are reviewed. The magnitude of the problem of accidental death and disability is examined. An EMSS description is provided, as are the methods used in prior studies to develop and evaluate such systems.

691. Diamond, Norman J., et al. "Evaluation of an Emergency Department Observation Ward." JACEP 5 (January 1976): 29-31.

> This is a report of a project to evaluate the usefulness of an observation, or holding area, in the operation of the emergency department at Harbor General Hospital, Los Angeles County, California.

692. Dooley, Alfred, and Lucas, Bernard,G.B. "The Evaluation of Emergency Care: Development of a Quantitative Criterion." <u>Annals of the Royal College of Surgeons of England</u> 60 (November 1978): 451-56.

> A study of fatal traffic accidents which occurred in North Yorkshire from January 1974 to July 1976 was conducted, employing a technique for comparing proportions of immediate to later deaths.

693. Dwyer, William. "Criteria Evaluation of Emergency Room Medical Care." <u>Bulletin American College of Surgeons</u> 60 (September 1975): 10-15.

> The results of a survey developed and implemented by the New Jersey Committee on Trauma of the American College of Surgeons are presented. Emergency departments were evaluated on the basis of the American Medical Association categorization criteria of hospital emergency capabilities.

694. Eisenberg, Mickey S., and Bergner, Lawrence. "Paramedic Programs and Cardiac Mortality: Description of a Controlled Experiment." <u>Public Health Reports</u> 94 (January-February 1978): 80-84.

> In the study, which was prospective and covered thirty months, cardiac mortality from out-of-hospital cardiac arrest in a community of 293,000 population was compared before and after the initiation of a paramedic services. Two adjacent communities, one with paramedic services, and one without, acted as controls. All three communities were similar with respect to age, sex, race, and incidence of out-of-hospital cardiac arrest. (Author's Abstract)

695. Eisenberg, Mickey S., et al. "Evaluation of Paramedic Programs Using Outcomes of Prehospital Resuscitation for Cardiac Arrest." JACEP 8 (November 1979): 458-61.

> Two evaluation methods, one statistical and one comparative, were developed to assess the effectiveness of paramedic programs in King County, Washington. The outcome of hospital admission following prehospital cardiac arrest was used as a measure of effectiveness. In the statistical method, actual outcomes were compared with predicted outcomes. In the comparative method, outcomes were compared with a standard in an adjacent community. Both evaluation methods are easily implemented. (Author's Abbreviated Abstract)

696. _____. "Paramedic Programs and Out-of-Hospital Cardiac Arrest. I. Factors Associated with Successful Resuscitation." <u>American Journal of Public Health</u> 69 (January 1979): 30-38.

> As part of an evaluation of whether the addition of paramedic services can reduce mortality from out-of-hospital cardiac arrest compared to previously existing emergency medical technician services, factors associated with successful resuscitation were studied. A surveillance system was established to identify cardiac arrest patients receiving emergency care and to collect pertinent information associated with the resuscitation. Outcomes, death, admission, and discharge were compared in two areas with different types of prehospital emergency care, basic EMT services versus paramedic services. (Abbreviated Author's Abstract)

697. _____. "Paramedic Programs and Out-of-Hospital Cardiac Arrest. II. Impact on Community Mortality." <u>American Journal of Public Health</u> 69 (January 1979): 39-42.

> Out-of-hospital cardiac arrest was studied in suburban King County, Washington, in an attempt to determine the impact of paramedic services on community cardiac mortality. A portion of the study area received paramedic services and the remainder received basic EMT services. A surveillance system identified all prehospital cardiac arrest incidents. The etiology and outcome were determined. Deaths due to primary heart disease were compared to community cardiac mortality figures for the same period of time and in the paramedic and EMT areas. (Abbreviated Authors' Abstract)

Literature

698. Frazier, William H., and Cannon, Joseph F. Experimental Health Delivery System: Emergency Medical Technician Performance Evaluation: Final Report. New Haven, Conn.: New Haven Health Care, May 1977. 255 p. (NTIS PB-272 379)

   An evaluation was conducted of the diagnostic accuracy and treatment appropriateness of EMTs in caring for 4,455 consecutive patients during a four and one-half month period. Data on EMT diagnosis and treatment and physician diagnosis were collected, and EMT data validated by observers. There were fifty-eight diagnostic conditions for which treatments were mandated as determined by a physician panel, affecting 2,233 (50 percent) patients. EMT diagnosis accuracy was measured using physician diagnosis as the standard, and rates of appropriate treatment were based upon the list of mandated treatments. Diagnostic accuracy tended to be mediocre, but treatment appropriateness varied by diagnosis and severity. Serious medical and trauma conditions received appropriate treatment far more frequently than nonserious conditions. Essential changes in educational approach and emphasis are discussed.

699. Geomet, Inc. Impact Evaluation of Emergency Medical Services Projects. 4 vols. Gaithesburg, Md.: July 1975. (NTIS PB-247-436/439)

   The report describes the five EMS demonstration projects which have been supported by the Division of Emergency Medical Services, Department of Health, Education and Welfare, since July 1972. Project target area include Arkansas, Illinois, eight counties in southern California, and seven counties in southeast Ohio. The purpose of the analysis is to evaluate the results of those demonstration projects and to assess the impact of their results upon current EMS activities. The objective is to explore the experiences of the five demonstrations for useful guidance in the organization of EMS systems in other parts of the country through identifying factors in system development associated with accomplishments or deficiencies.

700. Gibson, Geoffrey. "Evaluative Criteria for Emergency Ambulance Systems." Social Science and Medicine Journal 7 (1973): 425-54.

   The author discusses the inadequacy of evaluation criteria which have been used to date in evaluating emergency ambulance services. The author suggests three classifications for ambulance service measures. Several dispositional criteria for evaluating hospitals are presented.

701. _____. "Guidelines for Research and Evaluation of Emergency Medical Services." Health Services Reports 89 (March-April 1974): 99-111.

   With the EMSS Act of 1973, research and evaluation are no longer a desirable by-product of federal funding, but rather a major precondition for initial awards and subsequent renewal. This paper outlines methodologies for baseline and ongoing evaluation and commends their use by program applicants under the 1973 EMSS Act. Gibson's model for baseline evaluation includes: resources (hospital and ambulance), patient needs data (as well as patient demand), and resource utilization. He suggests methodologies for collecting data and criteria for evaluating it. Outcome measures have been ignored; Gibson discusses the difficulties in doing outcome assessment, yet strongly recommends their inclusion and suggests several measures. Ongoing evaluation should employ experimental designs: to assess pre- and postintervention changes in a project and control area; to assess effects of specific interventions (e.g., training); and to assess exogenous goals set by a funding agency.

702. _____. 100 EMS Evaluation Measures. Los Angeles: Conference on Urban EMS Systems, March 1976. 14 p.

These evaluative measures have been chosen with several ends in mind. First, they are responsive to, and fully compliant with, DHEW's mandatory program requirement for independent evaluation. Second, they allow two major sets of comparisons: before and after intervention comparison for the EMS system under review, and comparisons between the EMS system under review and other EMS systems. Third, the measures contain some that are universalistic in that they have and will be applied to all EMS systems, and some that are uniquely responsive to particular program needs. Fourth, the evaluative measures and their application will force EMS system managers through several consensus-producing discussions so that the evaluative activity will not only generate an agreement in current deficiencies, but on future program directions. Fifth, the measures have been chosen to exploit fully the present availability of EMS program data. Some new primary data collection will be necessary for certain measures not otherwise applicable.

703. Hannan, Edward L. "An Analysis and Evaluation of Emergency Services Holding Units." Ph.D. dissertation, Massachusetts University, Amherst Department of Industrial Engineering and Operations Research, June 1973. 209 p. (NTIS PB-250 576)

The purpose of the study is to develop a methodology for analyzing the needs for holding units as adjuncts to emergency service facilities, and for planning or modifying such units. The report begins with a discussion of the nature of holding units, their uses, and justifications. Methodologies are outlined for (1) comparing holding units, (2) evaluating the need for holding units, and (3) designing holding units. Each of these methodologies is applied to a specific situation.

704. Harber, T., and Lucas, B.G.B. "An Evaluation of Some Mechanical Resuscitators for Use in the Ambulance Service." Annals of the Royal College of Surgeons of England 62 (1980): 291-93.

Literature

This paper describes in detail the requirements for a mechanical resuscitator to be used in the ambulance service.

705. Headrick, R. Wayne, et al. "A Quality of Care Evaluation Measure for Emergency Medical Service Systems." Journal of Medical Systems 2 (1978): 281-301.

    This paper describes the development and validation of the System Input Severity Measure, which is composed of a set of single and multiple injury survival rates that would be expected to occur in a EMS system classified as providing baseline advanced life support services.

706. Holyfield, David, Jr., et al. Experimental Health Services Delivery Systems: Evaluation of Emergency Medical Technicians' Performance in Memphis, Tennessee. Memphis: Health Systems Management, November 1976. 45 p. (NTIS PB-272 217)

    This project's major goal was to develop and test a methodology which would allow for ongoing performance evaluation of emergency medical technicians. A modified encounter form was used to evaluate the ability of EMTs to assess correctly the patient's condition and to manage the prehospital patient according to mandated treatment protocols. The EMT indicated his clinical impression of the patient's condition on the encounter form, "checked off" appropriate blocks relating to assessment and management, and delivered the completed form to Emergency Department personnel who then made comments regarding the correctness/incorrectness of assessment and the appropriateness/inappropriateness of treatment. This information was recorded after the EMT had departed the ED. Analyses of encounters were made using an outside computer program as well as visual validation.

707. Huntley, Henry C. "How Effective Are Our Emergency Services?" Hospital Medical Staff 1 (February 1972): 1-10.

    Factors influencing the effectiveness of emergency medical services provided by hospital emergency departments and by ambulance services are considered. Lack of sufficient training of ambulance attendants and communications deficiencies between ambulances and hospitals are noted. It is suggested that it is the hospital's responsibility, through the emergency department, to train ambulance attendants as emergency medical technicians. The high cost of a well-equipped and well-manned ambulance service is discussed. It is suggested that one way to bring costs within reach is to employ emergency medical technicians on a full-time basis, assigning them jobs in the emergency department or elsewhere in the hospital between ambulance runs so that their special skills can be utilized fully.

708. Lanese, Richard R., and Keller, Martin D. Evaluation Studies. Southeast Ohio Emergency Medical Services Demonstration Project. Columbus: Ohio State University, Department of Preventive Medicine, 1976. 567 p. (NTIS PB-261 396)

Literature

The approach that was taken to the evaluation of the Southeast Ohio Emergency Medical Services Demonstration Project was generally that of evaluation as a social experiment. In this instance, the evaluation dealt with a health program specifically aimed at the provision of emergency medical services. In the evaluation of health programs or any social experiment, baseline information is obtained regarding the status of key variables before the program is underway. Consequently, the following six studies were undertaken: (1) resource and utilization data; (2) household interview surveys; (3) evaluation of trauma care; (4) simulation of the system; (5) evaluation of community education activities; and (6) communications component.

709. Larson, Richard C. "Approximating the Performance of Urban Emergency Medical Service Systems." Operations Research 23 (September-October 1975): 845.

Based on a hyercube queuing model, this paper presents a procedure for computing selected performance characteristics of an urban emergency medical service system. The model is intended for analyzing problems of vehicle location and response district design in urban EMS system.

710. Lauterbach, Stewart A., et al. "Evaluation of Cardiac Arrests Managed by Paramedics." JACEP 7 (October 1978): 355-57.

The effectiveness of cardiac resuscitations by Cincinnati paramedics was monitored for one year. The outcome of every arrest was assigned to one of four categories: dead on arrival, died in the emergency department, died in the hospital, or discharged alive, and each patient was followed until death or discharge from a hospital. Of the 147 people in the study group, 22 left the hospital alive, a long-term success rate of 15 percent, and another 26 percent died during hospitalization, 18 percent of the study population. This data is comparable to success rates reported by other prehospital care systems. Furthermore, this data indicates approximately 15 percent of people who have cardiac arrests outside of a hospital can survive through prompt intervention by trained personnel.

711. Leatherwood, Richard, et al. Assessment of Emergency Medical Systems Adequacy. 2 vols. Atlanta: Transaction Systems, September 1974. (NTIS PB-243 808)

This study reports on the adequacy of emergency medical services resources (ambulances, personnel, emergency departments, communication systems) by planning district within states, by state, by HEW region, and nationally. It also reports on the adequacy of private emergency medical services using a model to assess system adequacy. The results are presented in tabular form and narratively.

712. _____. Evaluation of Legal Barriers to EMS Implementation. 3 vols. Atlanta: Transaction Systems, November 1974. (NTIS PB-244 326; PB-243 725; PB-244 318)

Literature

The study examines how the absence or existence of state legislation encourages, facilitates, or impedes the provision of emergency medical services. Legislation for all states was analyzed with particular attention to the following areas: medical practice, paramedic training, responsibility for care, liability, licensure, vehicle codes, building codes, operation regulations, communications, public behavior, jurisdictional boundaries, fiscal responsibilities, and insurance. The report includes a catalogue of state legislation on EMS, tabular display of each state's legislation, display of potential legal barriers at state borders and display of status of legislation nationwide.

713. Lilja, G. Patrick, et al. "Clinical Assessment of Patients Undergoing CPR in the Emergency Department." JACEP 8 (February 1979): 81-83.

    To evaluate the effectiveness of long-term CPR, longer than an hour, an experiment was developed at North Memorial Medical Center and Hennepin County Medical Center, Minneapolis. Three patients who underwent long-term CPR are assessed. A mechanical cardiopulmonary resuscitator, Thumper, was used, together with invasive monitoring of pulse and blood pressure. Outcome of this project shows that patients undergoing long-term CPR are better managed by continuous blood pressure and pulse monitoring.

714. McCormick, John C., et al. "An Evaluation of a Model Ambulance Service." Paper presented at the American Public Health Association, Atlantic City, New Jersey, November 13, 1972. 18 p.

    This is an evaluation of the Freedom House Emergency Ambulance Service in Pittsburgh, Pennsylvania. Main findings are: (1) need for highly trained EMTs because of sufficient life-threatening emergencies; (2) high quality emergency medical treatment was provided; and (3) feasibility of using previously unskilled and underemployed persons and training them as EMTs.

715. McGibony, James T., et al. Jacksonville Emergency Medical Services Systems Outcome Measurement Research. Jacksonville, Fla.: Jacksonville Experimental Health Delivery Systems, December 1975. 375 p. (NTIS PB-251 607)

    Data were collected in the eight-county area for acute myocardial infarction (AMI), drug overdose, and accidents and injuries. Data for each patient were linked through ambulance, emergency room, and hospital, depending on patient entry. Investigations were conducted on effects of: (1) EMS on survival-mortality outcomes for AMI, overdose and accident and injuries; (2) EMS on cost, as a possible severity measures; and (3) various ambulance response and service on AMI mortality.

716. McNamara, John J., et al. "Assessing the Quality of Care by House Staff in a Municipal Hospital Emergency Department." JACEP 5 (April 1976): 257-61.

> The hypothesis that the results of process measures of the quality of care would be improved in a busy municipal hospital emergency department by using a medical record audit and reviewing findings with house staff and those responsible for their training was tested over a one-year period, and, tentatively, rejected. Out of twenty-one audit items, fourteen showed no significant change. Of the remaining seven, only three items showed significant improvement. Other mediating factors are related to quality of care in this setting such as patient-staff ratios, supervision, the focus of training programs, the physical plant, staff attitudes, behavior, and questions of control. (Author's Abstract)

717. McSwain, George R., et al. "Evaluation of Resuscitation from Cardiopulmonary Arrest by Paramedics." Annals of Emergency Medicine 9 (July 1980): 341-45.

> A series of one hundred consecutive victims of cardiopulmonary arrest were evaluated for treatment in the field by paramedic teams and for the patient's subsequent course. Analysis of the data correlated success rates with specific factors, including response, treatment, and transportation times, proximity to the emergency center, establishment of an intravenous line and administration of drugs, pulmonary aspiration of gastric contents, cardiopulmonary resuscitation by a bystander, cardiopulmonary arrest in the presence of the team, and other factors. Successful resuscitation was accomplished in 24 percent of cases, and 7 percent of the victims ultimately returned to their previous life-styles. (Authors' Abbreviated Abstract)

718. Mayer, Jonathan D. "Paramedic Response Time and Survival from Cardiac Arrest." Social Science and Medicine 13D (December 1979): 267-71.

> It has been assumed in the past that minimizing response time is an important goal in emergency medical services systems planning. However, this assumption has yet to be proven. In this analysis, 525 cardiac arrest cases are examined and the relationship between response time and survival determined. Paramedic response time is confirmed to be related statistically to long- and short-term survival from ventricular fibrillation. (Author's Abstract)

719. Methodologies for the Evaluation and Improvement of Emergency Medical Services Systems. 3 vols. Los Angeles: University of California, Division of Operations Research, August 1975. (NTIS PB-245 549/550/551)

> An efficient and general method of seeking an optimal deployment of emergency medical vehicles, in terms of minimizing the response time, is presented. The method combines a queuing model, an optimum seeking nonlinear algorithm, and

Literature

simulation. The queuing model is used to estimate a conditional mean response time for the given locations of hospitals and any initial set of locations of the emergency medical vehicles. The probabilities of one, two, and other emergency medical vehicles being busy, and hence increasing the mean response time, are estimated by simulation.

720. Mitchell, Janet B., et al. "Implications of Alternative Sampling Strategies for Emergency Medical Service Evaluation." Medical Care 17 (August 1978): 828-34.

> This paper studies four different sampling strategies and it measures their biases along three parameters of EMS system performance.

721. Mullner, Ross, and Goldberg, Jack. "An Evaluation of the Illinois Trauma System." Medical Care 16 (February 1978): 140-51.

> This article reports the assessment of the impact of the Illinois Trauma System in the southernmost region of the state. A four-year period was studied, 1970 through 1974.

722. _____. "Toward an Outcome-Oriented Medical Geography: An Evaluation of the Illinois Trauma/Emergency Medical Services Systems." Social Science and Medicine 12D (June 1978): 103-10.

> The purpose of the present study is threefold: to briefly review research by geographers working in health care services; to provide a description of the Illinois Trauma-Emergency Medical Services System; and to evaluate this system from a geographic perspective.

723. Ognibene, Margaret, et al. "The Time Relationship of Performance and Audit Feedback on Conformance with Emergency Department Process Criteria." Annals of Emergency Medicine 9 (March 1980): 123-25.

> Adherence to physician-developed process criteria is critical to the medical and legal acceptance of algorithm-directed nonphysician care of acute nonlife-threatening illnesses seen in the emergency department. It is generally assumed that adherence to prescribed medical process criteria results in acceptable patient outcomes. Changes in compliance with varying time delays in audit feedback and varying degree of supervision were evaluated. Evaluation indicated that, under ideal circumstances of daily audit and supervisory feedback, a conformance rate of 80 percent was achieved; thus, a 100 percent improvement over a group in which neither element was operative.

724. Pilcher, David B., et al. "Recurrent Themes in Ambulance Critique Review Sessions Over Eight Years." Journal of Trauma 19 (May 1979): 324-28.

> The value and benefit of regularly scheduled ambulance critique review sessions are discussed. The purpose of these sessions is to evaluate performance and review management of cases brought to the hospital by ambulance.

Literature

725. Pozen, Michael W., et al. "An Assessment of Emergency Medical Technician Performance as Related to Seasonal Population Influx." Journal of Community Health 3 (Spring 1978): 227-35.

> As people seasonally crowd resort areas, the demand for emergency medical services greatly increases. This study measured the impact of a threefold increase in Cape Cod's population during summer on the accuracy of emergency medical technicians' diagnoses and treatments. The study showed that the accuracy of EMT diagnosis rates is not apparently affected by seasonal population increase.

726. Rosenfeld, Leonard S., et al. Regional Emergency Medical Services in North Carolina: Monitoring and Evaluation. Chapel Hill: University of North Carolina, University Program in Health Services Evaluation, June 1974. 115 p.

> The focus of this work is upon the monitoring and evaluation of regional emergency medical services in North Carolina. There is an extensive review of the literature under the headings of: statistical systems, monitoring program evaluation, and research and evaluation.

727. Roy, A., et al. "Prospective vs. Retrospective Data for Evaluating Emergency Care: A Research Methodology." JACEP 8 (April 1979): 142-46.

> To overcome the lack of adequate data supplied by emergency department patient records for audit of quality of care, this project was developed at the Department of Emergency Medicine, University of Southern California, School of Medicine.

728. Sherman, Mark Alan. An Evaluation of the Effectiveness of Mobile Intensive Care Units in Reducing Deaths Due to Myocardial Infarction: Final Report. Evanston, Ill.: Northwestern University, June 1977. 299 p. (NTIS PB-271 380)

> Four communities which have introduced mobile intensive care units during the past five years were studied in this thesis. The independent variable was the presence or absence of a community-wide mobile intensive care system. The dependent variable was the mortality rate for acute myocardial infarction. The research design used was a multiple interrupted time series quasiexperiment. Data was obtained from hospital medical records. Analysis of the data showed a statistically significant decrease in mortality in two of the study communities. Plausible rival hypotheses were examined to see if factors other than the introduction of the mobile intensive care units (MICUs) could have led to the changes observed.

729. _____, et al. "Threats to the Validity of Emergency Medical Services Evaluation: A Case Study of Mobile Intensive Care Units." Medical Care 17 (February 1979): 127-37.

Literature

Much of the literature concerning emergency medical services evaluation has been criticized as unconvincing. Several sources of invalidity have comprised the interpretability of these studies. When true randomized experiments cannot be accomplished, quasiexperimental research designs offer greater interpretability than the more often used preexperimental designs. The paper describes eighteen threats to the validity of the evaluation, as well as the methods used for their control. (Author's Abstract)

730. Siler, Kenneth F. "Evaluation of Emergency Ambulance Characteristics under Several Criteria." Health Services Research 14 (Summer 1979): 160-76.

This paper outlines and analyzes a methodology for evaluating response time characteristics of emergency ambulance systems. The methodology is modeled after a Monte Carlo simulation technique and a heuristic optimal-seeking technique for locating emergency ambulances under several criteria based on response time distribution.

731. Webb, Duane D., and Lambrew, Costas T. "Evaluation of Physician Skills in Cardiopulmonary Resuscitation." JACEP 7 (November 1978): 387-89.

Thirty-five physicians were evaluated for performance skills in cardiopulmonary resuscitation according to standards of the American Heart Association. They were given instruction in only theoretical knowledge of CPR and a demonstration of the procedure, without supervised manikin practice. Only 22 percent of the physicians tested were able to compress and ventilate the manikin adequately in a simulated cardiac arrest.

732. White, Maria Salmon, and Gibson, Geoffrey. "Evaluation of an Emergency Department Patient Advocacy Program." JACEP 7 (April 1978): 145-48.

In the Patient Advocacy Program of the Adult Emergency Department of Johns Hopkins Hospital, first-year medical and health associate students provide patient teaching, crisis intervention, emotional support, assistance in patient-provider-family communication, resource referrals, information, and assistance in maintaining patients' rights. The advocacy program was evaluated through a three-month trial of a control group, patient advocacy group, halo group, and placebo group, including 412 study subjects in all. It was hypothesized that patient's satisfaction, behavior, and knowledge would improve significantly as a result of the advocate's intervention in this order: patient advocacy, halo, placebo, and control. Patient interviews and medical records were used to assess the impact of patient advocacy. Results did not support the hypothesis of either improvement or the ranked order. Competition with traditional roles, identification of advocates with providers rather than patients, and placing the needs of the institution over patients were suggested as explanations for the advocacy program's failure.

Literature

733. Willemain, Thomas R. The Status of Performance Measures for Emergency Medical Services. Cambridge: Operations Research Center, Innovative Resource Planning in Urban Public Safety Systems, July 1974. 32 p. (Document No. TR-06-74)

> The author addresses the question of determining which measures are appropriate for evaluating performance of emergency care systems. Measures are divided into three classes: input, process, and outcome measures. Input measures are those which serve to measure the boundaries and components of a system. The author points out that this is a measure of system potential only and does not adequately measure system performance. Process measures evaluate system efficiency and can be useful in monitoring system performance if one accepts the value of an EMS system.

734. Willing, Paul R. Issue on Impact of Evaluation Studies on Policy. Silver Spring, Md.: Macro Systems, March 1974. 34 p. (NTIS PB-243-032)

> This study relates relevant evaluation research to policymaking and illustrates through an analysis of the studies the factors which result in high impact of this research on policymaking. The analysis describes nine factors which play roles in linking relevant evaluation research with policymaking.

J. DISASTER PLAN—MUTUAL AID

The system must have a plan to assure that it will be capable of providing emergency medical services in the system's service area during mass casualties, natural disasters, or national emergencies.

In order to ensure a total utilization of all available resources, personnel, and equipment in an area or region larger than the EMS system, systems must provide for the establishment of appropriate arrangements with other EMS systems or similar entities servicing neighboring areas for the provision of emergency medical services on a reciprocal basis where access to such service would be more appropriate and effective in terms of the service available, time, and distance.

735. Allenbaugh, Gerald E. "Radios Restore Order to Chaos." Hospitals 46 (16 January 1972): 60-65.

> During the Los Angeles earthquake of 9 February 1971, a communication system was vital to effective and coordinated disaster operations.

736. American College of Emergency Physicians. "The Role of the Emergency Physician in Mass Casualty-Disaster Management: A Position Paper." JACEP 5 (November 1976): 901-2.

Literature

The paper puts forward the position that physicians who practice emergency medicine are qualified to assume a primary role in all aspects of mass casualty-disaster management.

737. American Hospital Association. <u>Checklist for a Hospital Civil Disturbance Preparedness.</u> Chicago: 1968. 4 p.

> The booklet presents a procedure for determining the degree of a hospital's preparedness to deal with a castastrophic situation and the mass casualties that may result from a civil disturbance.

738. _____. <u>Principles of Disaster Planning for Hospitals.</u> Chicago: 1967. 42 p.

> The publication outlines a hospital emergency preparedness plan in all its phases, including equipment, personnel, and communications. Some elements of planning included are: fallout protection, expansion of bed capacity, evacuation and relocation, administration, space allocation, and special emergency units.

739. _____. <u>Readings in Disaster Preparedness for Hospitals.</u> Chicago: 1973. 127 p.

> This is a compilation of a series of articles which describes in detail disaster procedures developed by hospitals and shows how some hospitals have responded to community disasters.

740. American Nurses Association. <u>Emergency Health Preparedness and Your Nursing Service: An Action Program for Hospitals, Community Agencies, and Nursing Homes.</u> Publication no. NS-11. New York: 1968. 30 p.

> This is a set of guidelines for action; it includes a bibliography and a selected list of films as sources of more detailed information.

741. "Area Agencies Ensure Success of Disaster Drill." <u>Hospitals</u> 53 (16 October 1979): 109-10.

> Local, state, and federal agencies cooperated in a disaster drill in Salem County, New Jersey. This type of exercise requires a vast amount of planning and cooperation among participating entities.

742. Baer, Eva. "Civil Disorder: Mass Emergency of the 70's." <u>American Journal of Nursing</u> 70 (June 1972): 1072-76.

> Tear gas injuries, hostilities between demonstrators and counterdemonstrators in the emergency department, and the tension over anticipated confrontations are a few of the unique problems of civil disorder. The article narrates the experience of Beekman Downtown Hospital, New York, in dealing with major civil disorders.

Literature

743. Bose, Kamal. "Disaster Planning." <u>Nursing Journal of Singapore</u> 19 (July 1979): 26-27.

   This article focuses on the hospital aspect of readiness for disaster victims. The importance of triage as the most important phase of in-hospital management of disaster casualties is stressed.

744. DeMars, Michael L., et al. "Victim-Tracking Cards in a Community Disaster Drill." <u>Annals of Emergency Medicine</u> 9 (April 1980): 207-9.

   The experience in using victim-tracking cards to evaluate the effectiveness of triage during a disaster drill at Detroit-Wayne County Metropolitan Airport is described. Tracking cards are cards of different colors used to track (follow) the victim through Assistance Procedures.

745. "Disasters, Flying Squads, and Immediate Care." <u>British Medical Journal</u> 2 (20 October 1979): 973-75.

   If a jetliner were to crash in central London, up to five thousand victims could be expected. This article deals with that possible scenario and methods of successfully managing such a disaster situation.

746. "Emergency Care in Natural Disasters: Views of an International Seminar." <u>WHO Chronicle</u> 34 (March 1980): 96-100.

   This essay is the result of an international seminar that was held to promote the exchange of knowledge and experience concerning the delivery of health services in the wake of such natural disasters as cyclones, earthquakes, floods, and droughts.

747. Executive Office of the President. Office of Emergency Preparedness. <u>Federal Disaster Assistance Program Handbook</u>. Washington, D.C.: July 1972. 36 p. (OEP Circular 4000, 7C)

   This handbook deals mainly with assistance available after the president has declared a major disaster. However, many departments and agencies have statutory authorities which permit them to assist even when damages do not justify such a presidential declaration. Both types of assistance are discussed and outlined, along with eligibility requirements and procedures for state and local officials applying for federal assistance.

748. _____. <u>The National Plan for Emergency Preparedness</u>. Washington, D.C.: December 1964. 128 p.

   The document is intended to give federal officials an overview of the field of emergency preparedness. The plan describes the roles of the federal, state, and local agencies and the kind of planning that will lead into effective action when a disaster arises.

Literature

749. Fisher, Charles J., Jr. "Mobile Triage Team in a Community Disaster Plan." JACEP 6 (January 1977): 10-12.

> Experience has shown poor disaster planning, lack of adequate communications and the absence of an on-scene commander to be the common and recurring problems during disaster rescue efforts. A mobile on-scene triage team operating in Sacramento has demonstrated the following advantages: immediate access; mobility; coordinated evacuation, treatment, and disposition of mass casualty victims; control of facility overload; and appropriate initial disposition to definitive care facilities.

750. Gates, William H., et al. "Medical Assistance Teams for Disasters." Ohio State Medical Journal 75 (June 1979): 378-82.

> The greater Cincinnati area medical disaster teams, including their mode of operations and procedures, are explained in detail. Also included are training, methods of activation, and communication linkage.

751. Gay, John H. "Papal Crowds: Medical Challenge." Journal of the Iowa Medical Society 69 (November 1979): 925-26.

> This paper describes the emergency health care coverage provided for Pope John Paul II's visit to Des Moines.

752. Gay, William, and Chenault, William W. Improving Your Community's Emergency Response: An Introduction to Disaster Planning. McLean, Va.: Human Sciences Research, May 1973. 127 p. (NTIS AD-762 067)

> This manual describes local comprehensive preparedness planning in nontechnical language. The document is based on research findings and reported experience involving human behavior and organization in disaster. The presentation is geared to the nonprofessional reader and seeks to initiate him into a process of full-time, year-round planning to combat the multiple hazards which may threaten his community.

753. Gerace, R. V. "Role of Medical Teams in a Community Disaster Plan." Canadian Medical Association Journal 120 (21 April 1979): 923-28.

> The role of medical disaster teams in London, Ontario, is reevaluated after two mock disaster exercises. An on-site team of three emergency physicians was formed to coordinate the disaster teams. The role of triage teams sent from the hospital to the disaster area was assessed and disaster procedures were reviewed.

754. Holloway, Ronald M. "Medical Disaster Planning: I. Urban Areas." New York State Journal of Medicine 71 (1 March 1971): 591-95.

755. _____. "Medical Disaster Planning: II. New York City's Preparations." New York State Journal of Medicine 71 (15 March 1971): 692-94.

Disaster plans, with their medical component, were stimulated by the fear of a nuclear holocaust and the realities of natural disasters. Planning for disaster must be realistic in terms of available resources and personnel. The first of the two above-cited articles deal with planning for disasters in urban areas in general. The second deals with specific preparations for New York City.

756. _____, et al. "The EMS System and Disaster Planning: Some Observations." JACEP 7 (February 1978): 60-61.

    One of the fifteen components of the Emergency Medical Services Systems Act of 1973 is disaster planning. This should be the culmination of the establishment of other components. Theoretical and practical disaster plans are hard to prepare and positive results cannot be assured. New York has planned for multiple casualty incidents to care for victims of fires, explosions, and major transportation incidents. The authors posit the idea that the ability to handle a mass disaster could be the best assessment of an EMS system's effectiveness.

757. Huntley, Henry C. "Formula for Disaster Preparedness." Hospital Topics 45 (August 1967): 64-66.

    The author stresses the idea that planning and adequate training in communities will pay high dividends when a disaster occurs. The normal hospital supplies and routines are insufficient to meet major medical emergencies. The Packaged Disaster Hospital (PDH) and the Hospital Reserve Disaster Inventory (HRDI) programs are discussed.

758. "Is Your City Prepared for a Major Disaster?" Nation's Cities, May 1973, pp. 26-56.

    This special issue devotes sixteen articles and features to urban disaster preparedness.

759. Jacobs, Lenworth M., et al. "An Emergency Medical System Approach to Disaster Planning." Journal of Trauma 19 (March 1979): 157-62.

    This paper emphasizes the importance of emergency planning, especially in light of the increase in natural disasters and terrorist attacks. The major principles of disaster planning are initial medical response, staging at the scene, and hospital notification. The role of triage in disaster planning is also explained.

760. Kekki, Pertti. "The Operation of a Health Centre after a Catastrophe in Finland." Journal of the Royal College of General Practitioners 28 (May 1978): 298-301.

    This paper describes how a local health center in Lapau, Finland, managed the victims of that country's most disastrous peace-time accident: an ammunition factory explosion.

Literature

761. Klinghoffer, Max. "A Pre-Triage Plan for Mass Casualty Care." Occupational Health and Safety 47 (November-December 1978): 32-35.

    Chicago's O'Hare Airport's disaster readiness program is delineated. The plan is based on a two-phase pretriage program and coordination with Chicago Fire Department and Memorial Hospital of DuPage County.

762. Lin, Swee Keng. "Medical Organization for Mass Disaster." Nursing Journal of Singapore 19 (July 1979): 23-25, 40.

    In a talk given at the Symposium on Management of Mass Disaster, Singapore, the author explains his points of view on the requirements for an ideal disaster management plan.

763. Milholland, Arthur V., et al. "Development and Prospective Study of an Anatomical Index and an Acute Trauma Index." American Surgeon 45 (April 1979): 246-54.

    The article describes two indexes obtained on severely injured patients treated at the Maryland Institute for Emergency Medical Services; they are the Acute Trauma Index (ATI) and the Blunt Anatomical Index (BAI).

764. Neal, Mary V. Disaster Nursing Preparation: Report of a Pilot Project Conducted in Four Schools of Nursing and One Hospital Nursing Service. New York: National League of Nursing, 1963. 254 p.

    This is a report of a study undertaken to find adequate ways in which student nurses and personnel in a hospital nursing service can be trained to cope with medical disasters.

765. Oberlander, Rachel. "Medical Care on a Day in May." Hospitals 53 (1 November 1979): 131-32.

    During the Indianapolis 500-mile race, there is a high probability that a disaster might happen. If a mass emergency occurs, it will be managed by an emergency facility which is one of the most complete of its kind.

766. "Planning Guide for Emergency Health and Medical Services and Disaster Recovery Coordination." Nebraska State Medical Journal 55 (January 1970): 66-74.

    This is a recommended guide to city, county, and regional planning for emergency conditions of various magnitudes. The guide is based on the premise that an effective emergency medical service system organization requires a governmental administrative structure, professional complement, medical direction, and adequate supporting services.

767. Pons, Peter T., et al. "An Advanced Emergency Medical Care System at National Football League Games." Annals of Emergency Medicine 9 (April 1980): 203-6.

Literature

This paper describes an on-going system for emergency medical services at Denver's Mile High Stadium during Bronco games. There are three manned first-aid stations. The types of cases seen during the 1978 football season are discussed.

768. Rutherford, W.H. "Experience in the Accident and Emergency Department of the Royal Victoria Hospital with Patients From Civil Disturbances in Belfast 1969-1972, with a Review of Disasters in the United States." Injury 4 (February 1973): 189-99.

   In a period of three years the Royal Victoria Hospital, Belfast, used its disaster code on forty-seven occasions. Forty-two disasters occurred in the United Kingdom since the organization of the National Health Service. Reports of these disasters are analyzed and interfaced with the Royal Victoria Hospital experience.

769. Shaw, Robert. "Health Services in a Disaster: Lessons from the 1975 Vietnamese Evacuation." Military Medicine 144 (May 1979): 307-11.

   The author describes his experience in "Operation New Life," Vietnamese evacuation in 1975, and how the lessons learned then can be applied to any future civilian disaster situation.

770. Snook, R. "Medical Care at Accidents and Disasters." Injury 10 (August 1978): 14-21.

   In order to provide appropriate and rapid care to victims of accidents and disasters, a preexistent, efficient, and organized system is necessary.

771. Storer, Daniel L. "Disaster Planning: Communications." Ohio State Medical Journal 75 (June 1979): 401-2.

   The Medical Assistance Team (MAT) concept developed in the Cincinnati area is explained. The MAT is an essential part of the general disaster plan and helps to establish efficient medical triage and treatment of disaster victims.

772. U.S. Department of Defense. Office of Civil Defense. In Time of Emergency: A Citizen's Handbook on Nuclear Attack and Natural Disasters. Washington, D.C.: March 1968. 92 p. (Publication no. H-14)

   The booklet is intended to alert the general public to prepare for disasters. Past experience shows many lives can be saved if people train themselves to meet possible emergencies. Family preparedness for life in fallout shelters, protection against nuclear fallout, first aid, and community planning are discussed.

773. U.S. Public Health Service. Division of Emergency Health Services. Assembling Equipment in the Packaged Disaster Hospital. Washington, D.C.: 1966. 135 p. (PHS Publication no. 1071-F-14)

Literature

This book provides directions, written and with illustrations, to help medical technicians and other type of personnel to set up some items in the Packaged Disaster Hospital (PDH).

774. _____. Catalog and Guide for Distribution of Packaged Disaster Hospital Materials. Washington, D.C.: 1967. 171 p. (PHS Publication no. 1071-F-15A)

This is a ready reference source that lists supplies and equipment in the two hundred-bed Packaged Disaster Hospital. It is useful to anyone who will set up or operate a PDH.

775. _____. Checklist for Developing a Packaged Disaster Hospital. Washington, D.C.: 1968. 21 p. (PHS Publication no. 1071-F-16)

This questionnaire will help hospital managers and other community planners to develop a well-organized plan to make effective use of a PDH. All the suggested activities must be performed before an emergency arises.

776. _____. Community Emergency Health Preparedness. Washington, D.C.: 1964. 20 p. (PHS Publication no. 1071-A-2)

Disasters, natural and nonnatural, occur in the United States almost on a daily basis. These destroy life and property. It was proven again and again that communities can meet disasters better if adequate disaster planning and continuing preparation are made. This booklet will help a community to plan for medical care following a disaster.

777. _____. Community Emergency Health Manpower Planning. Washington, D.C.: 1964. 20 p. (PHS Publication no. 1071-1-1)

Adequate disaster planning and measures are vital if a community expects to handle a major emergency. This document presents material that emergency medical service planners can use to assess their manpower potential, make assignments, and provide essential training.

778. _____. Disaster Nursing Preparation in Basic Professional Programs. Washington, D.C.: 1965. 172 p. (PHS Publication no. 1071-D-5)

This is a report on the hospital nursing services prepared by the National League of Nursing. Its purpose is to improve nurses' preparation in the handling of medical emergencies during disasters.

779. _____. Emergency Health Services--Preparedness Checklist for Hospitals. Washington, D.C.: 1969. 4 p. (PHS Publication no. 1071-G-3)

780. _____. Emergency Health Services--Preparedness Checklist for Metropolitan Areas. Washington, D.C.: 1969. 6 p. (PHS Publication no. 1071-A-8)

Literature

781. _____. Emergency Health Services--Preparedness Checklist for States. Washington, D.C.: 1969. 6 p. (PHS Publication no. 1071-A-9)

> These above-cited publications are aids that can be used to develop disaster readiness plans and procedures. They will help to determine deficiencies and to assess state of readiness to deal with disasters.

782. _____. Emergency Medical Supplies: Hospital Reserve Disaster Inventory (HRDI). Washington, D.C.: 1969. 14 p.

> This booklet describes free HRDI medical supplies and their importance to community hospitals during disasters.

783. _____. Establishing the Packaged Disaster Hospital. Washington, D.C.: 1969. 50 p. (PHS Publication no. 1071-F-1)

> This is an aid to planning and implementation at the local level so that Packaged Disaster Hospital can be used effectively. These packages are stored in selected communities in affiliation with a local hospital. They contain hospital supplies, equipment, and pharmaceuticals packed for long-term storage.

784. _____. Hospital Planning for National Disaster. Washington, D.C.: 1968. (PHS Publication no. 1071-G-1)

> The Joint Commission on Accreditation of Hospitals requires an accredited institution to have a written plan for the care of mass casualties, plus a rehearsal of the plan twice a year. This publication describes the procedure to fulfill the JCAH criteria on disaster planning.

785. _____. Model Plan: Metropolitan Area Emergency Health Service. Washington, D.C.: 1968. 79 p. (PHS Publication no. 1071-A-7)

> The plan outlined is a model that shows how a metropolitan area in the United States might prepare to assure effective emergency medical services during major disasters.

786. _____. Natural Disaster Hospital: Component Listing and Storage Data. Washington, D.C.: 1968. 49 p. (PHS Publication no. 1071-F-18)

> Natural disaster hospitals are prepositioned in or near areas where natural disasters, floods, twisters, or other major emergencies are likely to occur. This publication lists items contained in those hospitals.

787. _____. Preparing the Hospital Plan for Emergencies. Washington, D.C.: 1967. 48 p. (PHS Publication no. 1071-G-2)

> This publication is a collection of reprints that deal with aspects of hospital preparation for disasters. Some of the areas covered are: fallout shelters, emergency operations, communications for disaster, and back-up equipment system.

Literature

788. _____. <u>The Role of Medicine for Emergency Preparedness.</u> Washington, D.C.: 1968. 63 p. (PHS Publication no. 1071-I-8)

    Emergency medical services during disaster are an important aspect of disaster planning. Advanced planning and organized preparation by communities are the only way to assure adequate and effective medical services during disasters.

789. Yates, D.W. "Major Disasters Surgical Triage." <u>British Journal of Hospital Medicine</u> 22 (October 1979): 323-25, 328.

    This paper describes the application of a triage system in a "civilian" disaster situation.

Appendix
REGIONAL CONSULTANTS AND STATE COORDINATORS FOR EMERGENCY MEDICAL SERVICES

REGION 1

Regional Health Administrator
Attn.: Regional Consultant for Emergency Medical Services
Government Center
Boston, Mass. 02203

Connecticut

Director of EMS
Department of Public Health
79 Elm Street
Hartford, Conn. 06115

Maine

Director, Emergency Medical Services
Bureau of Health
State Department of Health and Welfare
Augusta, Maine 04330

Massachusetts

Director, Office of Emergency Medical Services
Massachusetts Department of Public Health
80 Boylston Street
Boston, Mass. 02116

New Hampshire

Director, Emergency Medical Service
New Hampshire Division of Public Health
61 South Spring Street
Concord, N.H. 03301

Rhode Island

Director, Division of Emergency Medical Services
Rhode Island State Department of Health
Davis Street
Providence, R.I. 02903

Vermont

Director, Emergency Medical Services
Vermont State Health Department
113 Colchester Avenue
Burlington, Vt. 05401

REGION 2

Regional Health Administrator
Attn.: Regional Consultant for EMS
Federal Building
26 Federal Plaza
New York, N.Y. 10007

New Jersey

Director, EMS
State Department of Health
P.O. Box 1540
Trenton, N.J. 08625

New York

Director, EMS
New York State Department of Health
28 Essex Street
Albany, N.Y. 12206

Consultants and Coordinators

Puerto Rico

Deputy Secretary of Health
Commonwealth of Puerto Rico
San Juan, P.R. 00910

Virgin Islands

Administrator, EMS
Knud Hansen Memorial Hospital
St. Thomas, V.I.

REGION 3

Regional Health Administrator
Attn.: Regional Consultant for EMS
P.O. Box 13716
Philadelphia, Pa. 19101

District of Columbia

Director for Planning and State
Agency Affairs
1530 East Street, N.W.
Washington, D.C. 20004

Delaware

Division of Emergency Health Services
State Health Building
Capital Square
Dover, Del. 19101

Maryland

Division of Emergency Medical Services
Department of Health Mental Hygiene
Baltimore, Md. 21201

Pennsylvania

Pennsylvania State Department of Health
P.O. Box 90
Harrisburg, Pa. 17120

Virginia

Director, Division of Special Health
Service
State Health Department
109 Governor Street
Richmond, Va. 23219

West Virginia

State Department of Health
State Office Building
1800 Washington Street, E.
Charleston, W.Va. 25325

REGION 4

Regional Health Administrator
Attn.: Regional Consultant for EMS
50 Seventh Street, N.E.
Atlanta, Ga. 30323

Alabama

Director, EMS Section
Bureau of Facilities Construction
Alabama Department of Public Health
Montgomery, Ala. 36104

Florida

Administrator, EMS Section
Department of Health and Rehabilitation Services—Division of Health
P.O. Box 210
Jacksonville, Fla. 32201

Georgia

Medical Director, Emergency Health
Unit, Facilities and Institute Section
Division of Physical Health
47 Trinity Avenue, S.W.
Atlanta, Ga. 30334

Kentucky

Director, EMS
Department of Human Resources
275 East Main Street
Frankfort, Ky. 40601

Consultants and Coordinators

Mississippi

Supervisor, EMS
Mississippi State Board of Health
Felix J. Underwood Building
Jackson, Miss. 39205

North Carolina

Chief, EMS
Division of Facility Services
P.O. Box 12220
Raleigh, N.C. 27605

South Carolina

Director, Division of EMS
Department of Health and Environmental Control
2600 Bull Street
Columbia, S.C. 29201

Tennessee

Director, EMS
Tennessee Department of Public Health
Chest Disease Hospital
Ben Allen Road
Nashville, Tenn. 37219

REGION 5

Regional Health Administrator
Attn: Regional Consultant for EMS
300 South Wacker Street
Chicago, Ill. 60606

Illinois

Division Administrator, EMS and Highway Safety
535 West Jefferson
Springfield, Ill. 62706

Indiana

Executive Director, Indiana EMS Commission
State Office Building
Indianapolis, Ind. 46204

Michigan

Coordinator, EMS
Division of Health Facilities, Standards and Licensing
3500 North Michigan
Lansing, Mich. 48914

Minnesota

EMS Coordinator
Department of Health
University Campus
Minneapolis, Minn. 55440

Ohio

EMS Coordinator
State Department of Health
450 East Town Street
P.O. Box 118
Columbus, Ohio 43216

Wisconsin

Chief EMS
State Department of Health and Social Services
P.O. Box 309
Madison, Wis. 53701

REGION 6

Regional Health Administrator
Attn.: Regional Consultant for EMS
1114 Commerce Street
Dallas, Tex. 75202

Arkansas

Director, EMS
Arkansas State Health Department
4815 West Markham
Little Rock, Ark. 72201

Louisiana

Director, EMS
Louisiana Health and Human Resources Administration
333 Laurel Street
Baton Rouge, La. 70804

Consultants and Coordinators

New Mexico

Director, EMS
New Mexico State Department of Health and Social Services
P.O. Box 2348
PERA Building
Santa Fe, N.Mex. 87501

Oklahoma

Director, EMS
Oklahoma State Health Department
Northeast Tenth and Stonewall Streets
P.O. Box 53551
Oklahoma City, Okla. 73105

Texas

Director, Texas State Health Department
Emergency Medical Services
1100 West Forty-Ninth Street
Austin, Tex. 78756

REGION 7

Regional Health Administrator
Attn.: Regional Consultant for EMS
601 East Twelfth Street
Kansas City, Mo. 64106

Iowa

EMS Planner
Iowa State Department of Health
Lusac State Office Building
Des Moines, Iowa 50319

Kansas

Director, EMS
714 West Tenth Street
Topeka, Kans. 66612

Missouri

Director, EMS
Missouri Division of Health
P.O. Box 570
Jefferson City, Mo. 65101

Nebraska

Director, EMS
Nebraska State Department of Health
Room 709
1003 "O" Street
Lincoln, Nebr. 68508

REGION 8

Regional Health Administrator
Attn.: Regional Consultant for EMS
Federal Office Building
Nineteenth and South Streets
Denver, Colo. 80202

Colorado

Director of Public Health
4210 East Eleventh Avenue
Denver, Colo. 80220

Montana

Coordinator Emergency Health Planning
Laboratory Building
Helena, Mont. 59601

North Dakota

Director, EMS
North Dakota Department of Health
State Capitol Building
Bismarck, N.Dak. 57501

South Dakota

Director, EMS Program
South Dakota State Department of Health
Pierre, S. Dak. 58501

Utah

Coordinator, EMS
Utah State Division of Health
44 Medical Drive
Salt Lake City, Utah 84113

Consultants and Coordinators

Wyoming

Director, EMS
Wyoming State Health Department
State Office Building
Cheyenne, Wyo. 82001

REGION 9

Regional Health Administrator
Attn.: Regional Consultant for EMS
Federal Office Building
50 Filton Street
San Francisco, Calif. 94102

Arizona

EMS Division
Department of Public Safety
P.O. Box 6638
Phoenix, Ariz. 85005

California

Chief, EMS
744 "P" Street
Sacramento, Calif. 95814

Hawaii

Director of Health
State Department of Health
P.O. Box 3378
Honolulu, Hawaii 96801

Nevada

EMS Coordinator
Division of Health, Welfare and Rehabilitation
201 South Fall Street
Carson City, Nev. 89701

REGION 10

Regional Health Administrator
Attn.: Regional Consultant for EMS
Arcade Plaza Building
1321 Second Avenue
Seattle, Wash. 98101

Alaska

State Health Service Coordinator
Comprehensive Health Planning Office
Department of Health and Social Services
Pouch H
Juneau, Alaska 99801

Idaho

Special Assistant to the Governor
Emergency Health Services
Department of Environmental Community Services
State House
Boise, Idaho 83720

Oregon

Director, EMS
Oregon State Board of Health
P.O. Box 231
Portland, Oreg. 97297

Washington

Director, Division of Social and Health Services
Division of Health
EMS
P.O. Box 1788
Olympia, Wash. 98524

AUTHOR INDEX

This index includes all authors, editors, compilers, and other contributors to works cited in the text. References are to entry numbers and alphabetization is letter by letter.

A

Abrams, Jerome 647
Acai, Stephen A., Jr. 454
Achabal, Dale D. 360
Acton, Jan Paul 645
Adams, Audrey 155
Adgey, A.A. Jennifer 431
Afifi, M. 10
Agisim, Elliot 463, 501
Alber, Philip R. 648
Allen, David 363
Allenbaugh, Gerald E. 312, 735
Alongi, Sharon 241
Alvin, Susan L. 678
American College of Emergency Physicians 242, 736
American College of Surgeons 361
American College of Surgeons. Committee on Trauma 362
American Hospital Association 464, 646, 737-39
American Medical Association 243
American Medical Association. Commission of Emergency Medical Services 465
American Nurses Association 740
American Society of Anesthesiology 466
American Trauma Society 671
Ames, Seth 544
Anderson, Gail V. 679
Andreasson, Rune 62
Andrews, Robert B. 580
Anwar, Rebecca A.H. 244-45, 274
Areawide and Local Planning for Health Action 503

Arkansas Health Systems Foundation 672
Arthur Young and Co. 681
Ayers, W.R. 649

B

Bachrach, Peter 682
Baer, Eva 742
Bailey, Judith A. 566
Barber, Janet 61
Bascomb Associates 467-69
Batten, R.L. 57
Beaman, Wrex W. 313
Beasch, Evelyn 178
Bell, Colling E. 363
Bennett, Margaret Jane 246
Benson, Don M. 364, 470
Berger, Thomas S. 600
Berge, S. 390
Bergner, Lawrence 694
Birch, H. 650
Bird, Kenneth T. 325
Block, Frank E. 247
Blum, Marc S. 365, 683
Blum, Thomas H. 471
Bobb, Timothy 504
Bobo, Phillip K. 585
Bobzien, William III 505
Boldt, Ronald 366, 684
Bolt, W. David 489
Bose, Kamal 743
Bouzarth, William F. 314
Bovier, F. 685
Boyd, David R. 367, 472, 651-52
Brearley, Kenneth S. 341

Author Index

Bregande, Barbara J. 567
Brennen, Dennis 148
Brigham, Peter A. 586
Brooks, Robert 182
Brose, Richard A. 500
Buckley, Bob 145
Bureau of Health Planning and Resource Development 506
Burghart, Hans 437
Burney, Richard E. 507
Burns, C.M. 568
Burt, John M. 368

C

Caldwell, Peggy 248
Callon, Helen F. 615
Camden, John W. Intro.
Cameron, Margaret 420
Campbell, Donald A. 673
Cannon, Joseph F. 698
Caroline, Nancy L. 249
Carr, Bennie Lou 109
Casey, G.B. 82
Cayten, C. Gene 272, 302, 653, 686-87
Center for Hospital Management Engineering 508
Chaiken, Jan M. 369-71
Chan, Linda S. 548
Chance, Graham W. 616
Chayet, Neil L. Intro
Chenault, William W. 752
Chipman, Martin 509
Chi Systems 342
Cleven, Arlene 250
Cohen, Irving J. 49
Cohen, Susan 10
Cole, Linda 654, 688
Comprehensive Health Planning Agency of Southern Wisconsin 617
Comprehensive Health Planning Council of South Florida 315, 510
Comprehensive Health Planning Council of Southwestern Indiana 588
Computer Science Corp. 689
Connauphton, Dennis M. 40
Cooper, Carole 372
Cooper, Mary Ann 438
Corey, James F. 55
Cowan, George S.M. 511
Cowley, R. Adams 439, 569-70
Cox, Roy E., Jr. 172
Craig, Thomas J. 526
Cram, A.E. 512
Crampton, Richard S. 373, 421, 428
Criswell, Barbara 164

Cronin, Kathie 251
Cross, Ralph E., Jr. 473
Czachowski, Ralph E. 422

D

Dalen, James E. 252
Daley, Edward V. 690
Danto, Bruce L. 627
Davis, John H. 63, 647
Davison, Stephen M. 513
DeClaris, Nicholas 571
DeClement, Frederic A. 586
Deems, John Michael 374, 535
Delfasse, C. 516
DeMars, Michael L. 744
Diamond, Norman J. 691
Doeksen, Gerald A. 375
Dooley, Alfred 692
Drury, Colin G. 316
Dunlap and Associates 376
Dwyer, William 693
Dyer, N.H. 423

E

Edlich, Richard F. 589
Eisenberg, Mickey S. 124, 253, 694-97
Ellingson, H.V. 460
Ethridge, Barbara 179
Evans, Lynn 669
Evans, William 653
Executive Office of the President. Office of Emergency Preparedness 747-48

F

Fahey, M. 343
Farrington, Joseph D. 53, 255
Feck, Gerald 590
Felknor, Rhea 572
Fernandez-Caballero, Carlos 198, 515
Fick, John 150
Fikes, J.M. 397
Fincke, Mildred K. 256
Finn, Peter 377
First, Joan M. 675
Fischer, Ronald P. 573
Fisher, Charles J., Jr. 749
Fisher, Roy 67
Fitzgerald, Robert T. 75
Fitzsimmons, James Albert 378-79
Fletcher, J.R. 516
Flexer, Morton 440
Flint, Lewis M. 257
Ford, J. Daniel 474

Author Index

Forkosh, David S.   475
Fortuna, Joseph Amaceo   258
Franck, Evelyn A.   346
Frank, H.D.   424
Fraser, Claire L.   517
Frazier, William H.   628, 698
Frey, Charles F.   259
Fries, Brant E.   518

G

Gahn, Donald   521
Garret, C.W.   317
Garvin, John M.   344
Gates, William H.   345, 750
Gavette, J. William   519
Gay, John H.   751
Gay, William   752
Geolot, Denise   260
Geomet, Inc.   699
George, James E.   50-51, 128, 656
Gerace, R.V.   753
Gettinger, C. Earl   530
Ghodse, A. Hamid   629
Gibson, Geoffrey   380-81, 476-77, 520-21, 657, 700-702, 732
Gladstone, Robert J.   370
Godley, Carol   524
Gold, Marsha R.   522
Goldberg, Jack   578, 721-22
Goldfrank, Lewis   261
Governor's Emergency Medical Services Advisory Council. Facility Task Force. State of Iowa   478
Graven, Stanley N.   626
Graves, Harris B.   523
Gray, Lois   524
Greensher, Joseph   607
Grenvid, Ake   262
Grigg, Thomas R.   263
Grottenthaler, Joel   576
Grundy, Betty L.   318
Gunderson, Harold   41
Gustafson, David H.   658
Gustafson, Gerald E.   319
Gutberlet, Ronald   621

H

Hacen, H.J.   602
Hackel, Alvin   618
Haeck, William T.   264
Haedtler, David R.   311
Hall, David S.   401
Hall, William K.   382-83

Hamilton, William F.   11
Hampton, Oscar P., Jr.   479-82
Hannan, Edward   525, 703
Hannas, Ralston R.   265
Harber, T.   704
Harrison, Elizabeth A.   12-22
Harrison, Robert R.   266
Hart, Joan   47
Harvey, John Collins   483
Haynes, B.W.   575
Hayter, Jean   591
Hea, Monique   159
Headrick, R. Wayne   705
Heidt, Robert S.   637
Heinzelman, Linda   120
Henry, William J.   320
Herrera, Alfredo J.   619
Herrmann, Nira   659
Hisserich, John Charles   384
Hoey, John R.   552
Hogan, Michael H.   245
Holloway, Ronald M.   385, 754-56
Holyfield, David, Jr.   706
Hood, Paul C.   134
Horobo, Roberta Gatjen   620
Horty, John F.   484
Houston, Gloria   177
Hubinger, John   116
Huddleston, William C.   630
Hudson, Nancy   151
Huffine, Carol L.   526
Huntley, Henry C.   707, 757

I

Iserson, Kenneth V.   267

J

Jacobs, Arthur R.   527
Jacobs, Lee   418
Jacobs, Lenworth M.   759
James, J.E.   131
Jarmon, Robert G.   321
Javis, James P.   386
Jayne, Harold A.   268
Jelenko, Carl III   387
Jelenko, Judith M.   387
Jenkins, Wayne   70
Jensen, Ken E.   388
Jessen, K.   442
Johnson, Graham   161
Jonas, Steven   528
Jones, Susan L.   529
Jordan, Robert F., Jr.   443
Josephson, Gordon W.   631
Josey, James Larry   444

Author Index

K

Kansas City. Area Hospital Association 485
Kanwit, John H. 530
Karas, Stephen, Jr. 531
Kaufman, Theodore 660
Keefe, Joyce 54
Kekki, Pertti 760
Keller, Geraldine B. 322
Keller, Martin D. 708
Kelman, Howard R. 532
Kentucky. State Department of Health 389
Keogh, Julian 592
Kiefer, Joseph N. 269
Kleiner, Betty 64
Klinghoffer, Max 761
Klippel, Allen P. 273, 486
Kolsters, W. 426
Korttila, K. 429
Krasnoff, Sidney O. 593
Krass, M.E. 488
Kresojevich, Ralph 533
Krischer, Jeffrey P. 661
Krome, Ronald 270, 534
Kvalseth, Tarald O. 535

L

Lambert, Susan 107
Lambrew, Costas T. 271, 323, 613, 731
Landau, Thomas 487
Landers, Gary A. 536
Lane, Dorothy 532
Lanese, Richard R. 708
Lanoy, M. 390
Larsen, Kenneth T. 537
Larson, Richard C. 346, 371, 392, 709
Lauro, Albert J. 275
Lauterbach, Stewart A. 710
Lazner, J. 393
Leatherwood, Richard 711-12
LeBlanc, Don 87
Ledger, Martha 272
Lee, Sung R. 273
LeTourneau, Barbara 538
Levalley, Norma 394
Levinson, Louis 154
Levy, Richard 274
Lewis, James E. 555
Lewis, Richard P. 425
Lilja, G. Patrick 713
Limmer, Allan N. 456
Lin, Swee Keng 762

Lohrisch, David Niven 539
Los Angeles. City Fire Department 395
Lowry, Frank 88
Lowry, Jon W. 275
Lucas, Bernard G.B. 692, 704
Luger, G.W. 426
Lund, Ivar 396

M

Maatsch, Jack L. 276
MacCally, Michael 277
McClendon, E.L. 397
McCormick, John C. 714
McDermott, Steve 324
McElroy, Charles R. 288
McGibony, James T. 715
Mackenzie, Colin F. 445
McKinley, Joe C. 594
MacMahon, A.G. 427
McManus, William F. 347
McNamara, John J. 716
McNeil, Delman 72
McSwain, Charlene 278
McSwain, Norman E., Jr. 35, 279, 296
Maddox, Darrell 574
Maher, Angela 77
Mains, Kenneth D. 280
Malone, Jim 94
Mangold, Karl G. 259, 281
Manning, Beatrice 540
Mannon, James M. 541
Marcus, Howard 428
Mariano, John P. 314
Mattox, Kenneth L. 542
Mattson, Joel L. 282
Maull, Kimball I. 266, 575
Maxwell, David M. 665
Mayberry, J.P. 488
Mayer, Jonathan D. 348-49, 718
Mazzi, Eduardo 621-23
Melenson, Richard S. 446
Menkes, Larry 129
Meyer, John W. 398
Meyer, Paul R., Jr. 603
Michaels, Harvey G. 499
Micik, Sylvia 608-9
Mid-Coast Comprehensive Health Planning Association 350
Mid-South Center Council for Comprehensive Health Planning 351
Milholland, Arthur V. 763
Miller, Kathryn P. 344
Miller, Sheldon I. 562

Author Index

Mills, John 283
Minerd, Rick 44
Mitchell, Janet B. 720
Moerkirk, George E. 576
Mofeson, Howard C. 607
Monroe, Charles B. 352
Morando, Rocco 284
More, G. 577
Moriatry, Richard W. 610
Moylan, Joseph A. 447
Moynihan, Barbara 628
Mullner, Ross 578, 721-22
Murphy, Ginger 167
Murphy, Raymond L.H. 325
Murphy, Steven P. 399
Murtomaa, Markku 429
Myrick, Justin A. 285

N

Nadler, Arnold David 353
Nagel, Eugene I. 326-27
National Academy of Sciences-National Research Council. Division of Medical Sciences. Committee on Emergency Medical Services 400
National Emergency Medical Services Information Clearinghouse 354, 676
National Highway Traffic Safety Administration (DOT) 328-29
National Library of Medicine 23
National Maritime Research Center 330
Neal, Marie 595
Neal, Mary V. 764
Neumann, Edward S. 448
Noble, John H., Jr. 24
North Shore Health Planning Council 355
Novack, Margit 638
Nowicki, Swan 78
Nussenfeld, Sidney 430
Nutt, Paul Charles 639

O

Oberlander, Rachel 765
Office of Telecommunications Policy 331
Ognibene, Margaret 723
Olsen, Michael P. 124
O'Neill, Brian 662
Otterbein, Scott A. 198
Owen, Wallace 190
Owens, Susan R. 543

Oxer, H.F. 449

P

Padget, Virginia 25
Paetow, Paul F. 640
Page, James O. 60, 286, 634-35
Pantridge, J. Frank 431
Parker, Frank E. 450
Parker, Jim 102
Peden, Guy T. 451
Penterman, Daniel G. 332
Perkin, N.E. 39
Perrine, Edward L. 401, 489
Perry, Charles 144, 186
Perry, I.C. 452
Pettet, Gary 453
Pilcher, David B. 724
Pizzi, Walter F. 287
Plaas, Hyrum 26
Plant, Janet 544
Pons, Peter T. 767
Pozen, Michael W. 46, 402, 545, 725
Praise, Israel 596
Pratt, Franklin D. 288
Proctor, Herbert J. 454
Pyo, Yoon H. 432

R

Raffensperger, John C. 603
Raming, Nancy D. 673
Recht, J.L. 36
Redmond, James M. 490
Reed, William E. 27-28
Region Three Health Planning Council 546
ReVelle, Charles 413
Riskin, Wayne G. 551
Robertson, William O. 611
Robortella, John 84
Romano, Teresa L. 289-92
Rosati, Robert A. 664
Rosen, Pet 547
Rosenberg, Robert G. 522
Rosenfeld, Leonard S. 726
Rossi, E.A. 624
Roussi, C.C. 665
Roy, A. 727
Rukavina, John 188
Rumage, William T. 641
Rutherford, W.H. 768

S

Sadler, Alfred M. 507

Author Index

Safar, Peter   403, 470
Samuels, Allen   455
Sandifer, Calvin R.   333
Sandler, Alan P.   548
Sandler, R.   356, 577
Scanlan, Elizabeth   570
Scanlan, Larry   405
Scherz, Robert G.   611
Schiro, Samuel George   316
Schneider, Jerry B.   406
Schnitker, Maurice A.   491
Schoeman, Milton E.F.   360
Schroeder, Oliver G., Jr.   642
Schwartz, George R.   666
Schwentker, Edwards P.   604
Scott, David W.   407
Scott, John E.   293
Shabazian, Dawn   294
Shavlik, Gerald   359
Shaw, Robert   769
Shearman, David J.   456
Shelby, Jones W.   549
Shepherd, Clovis   267
Sherman, Mark Alan   433-34, 728-29
Shiver, J.M.   550
Shoennken, William C.   42
Shubin, Herbert   583
Siler, Kenneth F.   334, 408, 730
Silva. Yvan J.   270
Silverston, Paul P.   295, 357-58
Singleton, Sharla   540
Skelton, Mary Beth   296
Skogman, David P.   457
Skulberg, Andreas   396
Slay, Larry E.   551
Smalley, Harold E.   335, 409
Smith, J. Stanley   492
Smith, Leslie R.   297
Smith, Vicki   176
Snook, R.   770
Sopp, Beverly   142
Sourwine, R.E.   298
Southeast Arkansas Economic Development District   632
Southern Maine Comprehensive Health Association   336
Sparacino, Sharon H.   643
Spitz, Louis   299
Spruill, Wade   108
Stafford, Valerie G.   300
Stanford Research Institute   458
Staroscik, Rudolf   302
Staub, Gerald F.   625
Stavas, E.S.   404
Steele, Richard   667
Steinmetz, Nicholas   552
Stensrud, Richard L.   459

Stevenson, Keith Allister   392, 410
Stone, Linda S.   683
Storer, Daniel L.   771
Stratmann, William C.   553, 644
Sudersanam, Vijay R.   110
Superior California Comprehensive Health System   677
Swoveland, C.D.   411
Symons, John G., Jr.   406

T

Taubenhaus, Leon J.   303-4
Taylor, Blaine   581
Taylor, Dianne P.   305
Tell, Robert   493
Temple, Anthony R.   612
Teufel, William   582
Texas. Municipal League   412
Thilliander, Brian D.   598
Thomas, J. William   554, 686
Thompson, C. Thomas   555
Thompson, R.G.   435
Thurber, Christine   519
Toregas, Constantine   413
Torrey, E. Fuller   414
Trunkey, Donald D.   582
Turner, H.S.   460
Tye, J.B.   306, 512

U

Uhley, Herman N.   337
Ullman, Ralph   553, 556-57, 644
U.S. Department of Defense. Office of Civil Defense   772
U.S. Department of Health, Education and Welfare. Division of Emergency Health Services   29
U.S. Department of Health, Education and Welfare. Division of Emergency Medical Services   494, 688
U.S. Department of Transportation. National Highway Traffic Safety. Committee on Ambulance Design Criteria   415
U.S. Department of Transportation. National Highway Traffic Safety Administration. Office of Administrative Services   32
U.S. Department of Transportation. National Traffic Safety Administration. Office of Management Systems   33
U.S. General Services Administration. Federal Supply Service. General Services Administration   416

Author Index

U.S. Public Health Service. Division of Emergency Health Services 773-88

V

Valbona, Carlos 669
Vander Veer, Joseph 166
Vaughn, Byron 558
Veltri, Joseph C. 612
Virginia. Polytechnic Institute and State University 338
Vogt, Fred B. 339
Volz, Richard A. 417
Voorman, Dorothy M. 56

W

Waekerle, Joseph F. 307
Wagner, Mary M. 599
Walker, Lynn Levi 559-62
Walker, William 471
Waller, Julian A. 418, 495-96
Waltz, Robert C. 497
Watkins, Richard N. 308
Watts, Richard W. 432
Webb, Duane D. 731
Weber, Lodge L. 58, 138
Weigel, J.A. 364
Weil, Max Harry 583
Weiner, Mary Anne 309
Weiss, Toni 86
Welch, Benjamin 461

Wenzel, V. 670
Werner, Martin 340
West, Irvan M. 419
Weston, P.A.M. 584
Wetzel, Thomas 65, 105
Wheeler, E. Todd 614
White, Maria Salmon 732
White, Roger D. 310
Willemain, Thomas R. 498-99, 733
William, B.T. 563
William, Thomas J. 11
Williams, Phyllis M. 359
Willing, Paul R. 734
Wilson, Frank P. 564
Wingert, Willis 565
Wiseley, Sally F. 605
Witt, Richard C. 311
Wolff, Peter 377
Woll, Myra 501
Wood, A. Michael 462
Wright, Peter 340

Y

Yates, D.W. 789
Youmans, Roger L. 500
Young, Steven R. 598

Z

Zachman, Richard D. 626
Zenz, Carl 68
Zimberg, Sheldon 633
Zschoche, Donna 43

TITLE INDEX

This index includes all titles of books and published papers and pamphlets cited in the text. References are to entry numbers and alphabetization is letter by letter.

A

Air Medical Evacuation System (AMES) Demonstration Project 436
Allocation of Emergency Units 369
All Shortest Distances in Large Serial Networks 368
Ambulance 416
Ambulance Placement Strategies for Emergency Medical Systems (Blum) 365
Ambulance Placement Strategies for Emergency Medical Systems (Smalley) 409
Ambulance Service in Texas 412
Ambulance Service in Vermont 418
Analysis of Ambulance Service Needs in Yuba-Sutter Counties 366, 684
Analysis of Burn Care Services and Needs in Southwestern Indiana with Conclusion and Recommendations 588
Assembling Equipment in the Packaged Disaster Hospital 773
Assessment of Emergency Medical Systems Adequacy 711
Assessment of the Kinds of Measures (and their Availability) Required to Determine the Impact of Categorization on Hospital Finance, An 467

B

Bibliography of Emergency Medical Services Literature Obtained from Computer Indexed Information Sources 9
Biotelemetry 12

C

Catalog and Guide for Distribution of Packaged Disaster Hospital Materials 774
Categorization of Emergency Room Facilities in Northeastern Kentucky 489
Categorization of Emergency Services 485
Categorization of Hospital Emergency Capabilities 465
Categorization of Hospital Emergency Services: Report of a Conference 464
Categorization of Hospital Emergency Services: Selected Bibliography 30
Central California M.A.S.T. Program--Military Assistance to Safety and Traffic 350
Checklist for a Hospital Civil Disturbance Preparedness 737
Checklist for Developing a Packaged Disaster Hospital 775
Communications Guidelines for Emergency Medical Services 328
Communications Plan for Emergency Medical Systems 313
Community Emergency Health Manpower Planning 777
Community Emergency Health Preparedness 776

Title Index

Considerations Which Are Relevant to the Methodology for Measuring the Financial Impact of Categorization 468

Consumer Information and Education Handbook for the Emergency Medical Services System 672

Coverage Models of Emergency Facilities Categorization 499

Critical Care Seminar Prospectus Emergency Cardiac Care 613

D

Data Protiles EMS Public Awareness and Utilization Patterns in Arkansas 675

Demand for Health Care Among the Urban Poor with Special Emphasis on the Role of Time 645

Description and Analysis of Eighteen Proven Emergency Ambulance Service Systems 372

DeSoto County Emergency Medical Service Transportation Plan 351

Development and Application of a Methodology for Reviewing Areas of the County Where Categorization Is Claimed to Have Taken Place 469

Development and Application of a Planning Methodology to Increase the Effectiveness of the Emergency Medical Transportation System for the Southern Maine Comprehensive Health Association 342

Development of a Minimum Data Set for Emergency Medical Services Patient Recordkeeping 667

Disaster Nursing Preparation 764

Disaster Nursing Preparation in Basic Professional Programs 778

Dispatcher Emergency Medical Technician Training Course 329

Dispatching the Units of Emergency Services Systems Using Automatic Vehicle Location 346

E

Economics of Highway Emergency Ambulance Service 376

Economics of Rural Ambulance in the Great Plains 375

Effective Company Command for Company Officers in the Professional Fire Service 286

Emergency Ambulance Service in Kentucky 389

Emergency Care Bibliography 10

Emergency Care Capabilities of Wisconsin Hospitals 463

Emergency Care of the Critically Ill Newborn Infant 620

Emergency Care Quality 669

Emergency Health Preparedness and Your Nursing Service 740

Emergency Health Services-- Preparedness Checklist for Hospitals 779

Emergency Health Services-- Preparedness Checklist for Metropolitan Areas 780

Emergency Health Services-- Preparedness Checklist for States 781

Emergency Health Services Selected Bibliography 29

Emergency Health System Planning 11

Emergency Medical Communications, Wisconsin 1969 340

Emergency Medical Services Intro.

Emergency Medical Services: A Bibliography with Abstracts 33

Emergency Medical Services: Costs 13

Emergency Medical Services: Health Planning 14

Emergency Medical Services: Hospitals 15

Emergency Medical Services: Rural Areas 16

Emergency Medical Services: Selected Bibliography 24

Emergency Medical Services: Transportation 17

Emergency Medical Services: Transportation Guidelines 354

Emergency Medical Services: Utilizationa 18

Emergency Medical Services and Care 19

Emergency Medical Services and Neighborhood Health Centers 524

Emergency Medical Services Audiovisuals 198

Emergency Medical Services Bibliography 25

Emergency Medical Services Communications 338

Emergency Medical Services for Fire Departments 634

Title Index

Emergency Medical Services Public Education Guidebook 676
Emergency Medical Services Public Information Manual 671
Emergency Medical Services Systems Program Guidelines, The p. 4
Emergency Medical Supplies 782
Emergency Medical Technician Instructor Training Institute 250
Emergency Medical Transportation 355
Emergency Rescue Ambulance Deployment Project 395
Emergency System Simulator (ESSIM) 554
Emergency Room Utilization: Overview and Implications 504
Emergency Room Utilization at Day Kimball Hospital 540
Emergency Room Utilization in Central New York 503
Emergency Services: The Hospital Emergency Department in an Emergency Care System 502
Emergency Telephone Number (911) 331
EMS Handbook for Patient Recordkeeping and List of Minimum Data 668
EMS Planning and Evaluation 686
EMS Transportation Overview 356
Establishing the Packaged Disaster Hospital 783
Evaluation Methodology for Emergency Medical Services Systems, An 689
Evaluation of Emergency Medical Services Systems Impact 683
Evaluation of Legal Barriers to EMS Implementation 712
Evaluation of Operations and Marginal Costs of MAST Alternatives 458
Evaluation of Policy Related Research in Emergency Medical Services, The 26
Evaluation of the Effectiveness of Emergency Medical Services Councils in Wisconsin 682
Evaluation of the Effectiveness of Mobile Intensive Care Units in Reducing Deaths Due to Myocardial Infarction, An 728
Evaluation Studies 708
Evaluation Workbook for EMS 681
Experimental Health Delivery System 698
Experimental Health Services Delivery Systems 706

Extension of Project CARE-SOM Coordinated Accident Rescue Endeavor, State of Mississippi 451

F

Feasibility Analysis for a Consolidated Emergency Trauma Center 577
Feasibility Study for the Development and Use of the Satellite Communications System to Provide Shipboard Emergency Medical Services 330
Federal Disaster Assistance Program Handbook 747

G

Goals and Guidelines for a System of Emergency Facilities for Dade County 510
Guide for a Workshop to Identify the Physician as the Key Figure for Improving Emergency Medical Services in the Community 242
Guidelines for Mobile Intensive Care Paramedics 423
Guidelines for Neo-Natal Intensive Care Units 617
Guidelines for Patient Record-Keeping Systems for Emergency Medical Service 650
Guidelines to Functional Programing, Equipping, and Designing Hospital Outpatient and Emergency Activities 506
Guide to Program Planning 243

H

Health Care Delivery 20
Health Services in Rural Areas 21
Helicopter Ambulance Service to Emergencies (HASTE) 441
Helicopters in Emergency Medical Services 450
Highway Safety Program Manual 690
Hospital Emergency Room, The 23
Hospital Emergency Services in Vermont 530
Hospital Planning for National Disaster 784

Title Index

I

Impact Evaluation of Emergency Medical Services Projects 699
Improving Emergency Services Through Community Involvement 638
Interim Study of Fort Wayne, Indiana Hospital's Emergency Room Utilization 546
In Time of Emergency 772
Irreducible Functions of the Hospital Emergency Room 532
Issue on Impact of Evaluation Studies on Policy 734

J

Jacksonville Emergency Medical Services Systems Outcome Measurement Research 715

L

Land Mobile Communication 27
Legal Implications of Emergency Care Intro.
Locating Ambulance Dispatch Centers in an Urban Region 406

M

Manual for Developing Community Programs, A 677
Medical Requirements for Ambulance Design and Equipment 400
Messages Received at an EMS Dispatching Center 322
Methodologies for the Evaluation and Improvement of Emergency Medical Services Systems 719
Methodologies for the Evaluation and Improvement of Emergency Medical Service Systems: Final Report 680
Methods for Allocating Urban Emergency Units 371
Military Assistance to Safety and Traffic (MAST) Procedural Guide 446
Military Assistance to Safety and Traffic (MAST) Operations Manual 455
Model Ordinance Regulating Ambulance Service 361
Model Plan 785

N

National Plan for Emergency Preparedness, The 748
Natural Disaster Hospital 786

O

Objectives of EMS Communications System 315
100 EMS Evaluation Measures 702
On Insensitivities in Urban Redistricting and Facility Location 392
Operational Aspects of Emergency Ambulance Service 410

P

Patient's Bill of Rights, A 646
Patterns of Utilization of the Emergency Room at Middlesex Memorial Hospital 543
Planning a Helicopter Transportation System to Augment Emergency and Regional Medical Programs in a Test Region of West Virginia 443
Planning the Efficient Delivery of Pre-Hospital Emergency Medical Services 353
Portable Radio Equipment 28
Preparing the Hospital Plan for Emergencies 787
Principles of Disaster Planning for Hospitals 738
Public Education and Information for Emergency Medical Services Development 673

R

Readings in Disaster Preparedness for Hospitals 739
Regional Emergency Medical Services in North Carolina 726
Report on a Program to Categorize Emergency Medical Service Facilities in Iowa Hospital 478
Response of Emergency Units 391
Role of Medicine for Emergency Preparedness 788
Rural Emergency Medical Services 31

S

Simple Procedure for the Allocation of Ambulances in Semi-Rural Areas, A 386

Title Index

Some Trends in the Delivery of Ambulance Services 370
Southeast Arkansas District Plan for the Prevention, Treatment, and Control of Alcohol Abuse and Alcoholism 632
Southern Main's Emergency Medical Communication System 336
Status of Performance Measures for Emergency Medical Services, The 733
Study of Emergency Room Utilization, A 508
Study of Three Small Upstate Emergency Departments 519
System Approach to the Care of the Trauma Victim, A 580
System Response to the Poisoned Patient 609
Systems Approach to the Care of the Burn Victim, A 597

T

Technical Reports of the National Highway Traffic Safety Administration 32
Telecommunications in Medicine 22
Telemetry and Physician-Rescue Personnel Communications 326
Telemetry Utilization for Emergency Medical Services System 335

U

Use of Helicopters for Air Delivery and Emergency 34
Utilization of a Psychiatric Nurse by the Staff of an Emergency Room, The 305

W

Wisconsin Emergency Department Utilization Study 501

SUBJECT INDEX

This index is alphabetized letter by letter and references are to entry numbers, unless preceded by a "p."

A

Academy of Health Sciences 192
Academy of Medicine (Cleveland) 497
ACT Foundation (Advanced Coronary Treatment) 200
Acute Trauma Index (ATI) 763
Africa, flying doctor service in 462. See also South Africa
Airports, disaster planning by 744-45, 761
Air transportation 353, 399, 419, 436-62, 465, 624
  bibliography on 34
  in burn care 586
  in rural areas 443, 448
  in spinal cord injury care 602
Alabama, regional burn care in 585
Alcoholics, emergency treatment of 533, 549, 630, 632-33
Alexandria Plan 264-65
Allegheny County, Pa., hospital emergency facilities in 470
Ambulance and Medical Services Association (AMSA) 201
Ambulance Dispatch Center Location (ADLOC) 406
Ambulance Law (Massachusetts, 1973) 355
Ambulance services 285, 348, 360-419, 475, 521, 568, 624
  bibliographies on 14, 18
  economic aspects 366, 375-76, 389, 397, 401-2, 404, 409-10, 684

fees 4
taxation 4
education and training for 284, 303, 310, 364, 385, 393, 405, 409, 419, 707, 714
equipment and design 354, 362, 389, 400, 403, 415-16, 704
evaluation and standards 380-81, 405, 409, 684, 700, 707, 711, 715, 717-19, 724, 730
fire department-based 364
law 387
  model ordinance 361
location, dispatch, allocation, and demand 263, 334, 353-54, 360, 363, 365, 369, 371, 374, 376, 378-79, 382-86, 391-92, 395, 405-9, 411, 413, 417, 554, 709, 718-19, 730
hospital-based 388
privately owned 355, 360
reporting forms for 670
rural 375, 386, 397-98, 401, 417, 419
volunteers serving on 364
See also Coronary care units, mobile; Intensive care units, mobile
Ambulatory care. See Outpatient services
Ambulatory Care Center-Emergency Services System (ACESS) 550
American Academy of Orthopaedic Surgeons 202
American Ambulance Association 203
American Association for the Surgery of Trauma 204, 361

173

Subject Index

American Association of Critical Care Nurses 205
American Association of Junior Colleges 243
American Association of Trauma Specialists 206
American Association of Trauma Specialists Education Foundation 207
American Board of Emergency Medicine 208
American Burn Association 209
American College of Emergency Physicians 210
　Residency Training Program in Emergency Medicine 265, 275
American College of Surgeons 211, 361
　Committee on Trauma 582, 693
American Heart Association 193, 230, 301, 731
American Hospital Association 195, 231, 464, 646
American Medical Association 194, 243
　hospital emergency room guidelines 463, 465, 469-70, 482, 486, 489, 493, 693
American National Red Cross 232, 301
American Public Health Association 233
American Society of Anesthesiology 500
American Trauma Society 212
Arkansas
　EMS evaluation in 699
　prevention and treatment of alcoholism in 632
　public awareness of EMS systems in 675
Associated Public Safety Communication Officers 234
Atlanta
　ambulance service in 409
　EMS communication systems in 335
　hospital emergency facility utilization in 535
Australia
　flying doctor service in 456
　prehospital trauma care in 343

B

Bacteriologists 262
Beekman Downtown Hospital (New York) 742

Behavioral emergencies 627-33. See also Alcoholics; Drug abuse; Psychiatry; Rape; Suicide
Biotelemetry, bibliography on 12
Blunt Anatomical Index (BAI) 763
Bronx Municipal Hospital Center 678
Brooke Army Medical Center, Emergency Services Section 551
Burn care 585-99
　planning and organization of 596
　regional programs for 585, 595
　rural 595
　triage in 589, 594
Burn Foundation of Greater Delaware Valley 213

C

California
　ambulance service in 366, 419, 684
　emergency helicopter services in 455
　EMS communication systems in 340
　EMS evaluation in 699
　health education in 677
　neonatal care in 620
California Emergency Department Nurses Association 248
California Military Assistance to Safety and Traffic Coordinating Committee 350
Canada
　ambulance services in 405
　development of regional trauma units in 568
Cardiac care units. See Coronary care units
Cardiopulmonary resuscitation 252-53, 278, 301, 373, 429, 643, 677, 713, 731
Central Connecticut State College 250
Central Indiana Emergency Medical Services Council 636
Charity Hospital (New Orleans) 275
Chicago
　disaster planning in 761
　health education and information in 674
　hospital emergency facilities in 474-75
　utilization studies 514
Chicago. Midwest Regional Spinal Injury Care System (MRSICS) 603
Chicago, University of. Hospital 547
Children
　neglect of 630
　poisoning of 607, 609, 611

174

Subject Index

Children's Hospital Medical Center (Boston) 522
Cincinnati, disaster planning in 750, 771
Cincinnati General Hospital 299
Cities. See Urban areas
Civil disorder. See Disaster planning and management
Cleveland, Ohio
 emergency coronary care in 432
 hospital emergency facilities in 497
Clinics 519-21
Columbia, Mo., EMS evaluation in 690
Columbus, Ohio, EMS system in 425
 communication aspects 322
Communications; telecommunications 312-40, 350, 385, 389, 409, 464-65, 510, 521, 542
 bibliographies on 9, 14, 19, 21-22, 24, 27-28
 education for 329
 evaluation of 707-8, 711-12
Computerized Ambulance Location Logic 378-79
Computers. See Models (mathematical and computer); Patient care, record keeping in
Cook County (III.) Hospital 514, 652
Coronary care units 613-14, 654
 admissions to 545
 bibliography on 17
 mobile 337, 373, 420-35
  rural 422, 428
  training for 423
 uniform reporting systems and evaluation of 655, 694-97, 710, 715, 717-18, 728
 standards and guidelines 301
 See also Electrocardiograms
Cowley, R. Adams 581
Critical care. See Behavioral emergencies; Burn care; Coronary care units; Infants, newborn; Intensive care units; Poisoning; Spinal cord injury; Trauma
Cyclones. See Disaster planning and management

D

Dade County, Fla.
 EMS communication system in 315
 hospital emergency facility utilization in 510

Day Kimball Hospital (Putman, Conn.) 540
Denver, Colo., emergency air transport in 453
Des Moines, Iowa, disaster planning in 751
DeSoto County, Miss., EMS transportation system in 351
Detroit
 ambulance service in 382-83
 hospital emergency services in 493
 utilization studies 533-34
Detroit General Hospital 533
Detroit-Wayne County Metropolitan Airport, disaster planning at 744
DeWitt Army Hospital 537
Disaster planning and management 509-10, 735-89
 bibliographies on 29, 740
 communications in 312, 735, 749-50, 787
 community EMS councils in 641
 national planning 748
 triage in 743-44, 749, 753, 759, 761, 771, 789
Domestic conflict 630
Droughts. See Disaster planning and management
Drug abuse 609, 629-30, 715

E

Earthquakes. See Disaster planning and management
Electrocardiograms, telemetric evaluation of 321, 323, 326, 337
Emergency Care Information Center 5, 196
Emergency Care Research Institute 214
Emergency Department Nurses Association 215
Emergency Medical Services Administrators Association 216
Emergency Medical Services Education 217
Emergency Medical Services Information Center (EMSIC) 5, p. 12, 197
Emergency Medical Services System Act (1973) pp. 1-2, 7, p. 31, 494, 521, 606, 608, 635, 681, 700, 756

Subject Index

Emergency medical services systems
administration, management and
organization pp. 1-2,
10, 16, 258
    study and teaching of 267,
272
    certification and standards 9
    consumer participation in 636-44,
682
    definition p. 1
    economic aspects (funding, costs,
etc.) 10, 11, 13, 16, 17,
    legislation 1-4
    manpower and training 9, 16,
241-311
    organizations involved with 200-
240
        directly 200-229
        government and official 230-35
        peripherally 236-40
    planning in 11, 16, 17
    review and evaluation of 9, 17,
678-734
    sources on 5-199
        audiovisual aids 192-99
        bibliographies 9-34
        computer data bases 6, 7,
p. 12
        information centers 5-8
        periodicals 35-191
            journals 35-77
            newsletters 77-191
    See also aspects of EMS (e.g.,
Communications; Disaster
planning and management;
Health education; Patient
care; Transportation)
Emergency medical technicians and
paramedics 271, 292,
687
    certification and standards p.4
255
    education and training p.4, 243,
247, 249, 253-55, 257,
266, 277, 284, 296-97,
302, 310, 357, 385, 393,
405, 409, 419, 423, 654,
707, 712, 714
        for communications 329
        instructor education 250
    evaluation of 694-98, 706, 710,
717-19, 725
    in intensive care units 262, 654-
55, 694-97, 710, 717-18
Emergency Medicine Foundation 218

Emergency Medicine Residents Association 219
Emergency Medicine Speciality Certification Examination (EMSCC)
276
Emergency System Simulator (ESSIM)
554
EMT Apprenticeship Program 220
England. See United Kingdom
Erie County, N.Y.
    ambulance service in 381
    EMS communication system in 316

F

Fairfax, Va., hospital emergency
facility utilization in 550
Fallout shelters 772, 787
Federal government, support for
ambulance services by 376
Finland
    disaster management in 760
    emergency coronary care in 429
Fire departments, emergency medical
services of 634-35
    personnel administration in 286
    transportation services in 354-55,
364
First aid
    bibliography on 29
    training for 251, 288
Floods. See Disaster planning and
management
Folk medicine, among Mexican Americans 548
Fort Wayne, Ind., hospital emergency
facility utilization in 546
Freedom House Emergency Ambulance
Service (Pittsburgh) 714

G

General Hospital (Norfolk, Va.) 598
General Hospital (Philadelphia) 688
Georgetown University. Pediatric
Pulmonary Program 649
Georgia
    ambulance law in 387
    emergency helicopter services in 446
Germany, West
    mobile intensive care units in 424,
437
    prehospital trauma care in 343
Golf carts, as EMS vehicles 354,
394
Good Samaritan Law 4

Subject Index

Government. See Federal government; State government
Great Britain. See United Kingdom
Greek Americans, EMS information sources for 674

H

Harbor General Hospital (Los Angeles) 691
Health centers, neighborhood
 bibliography on 18
 utilization of 522, 524
Health education 287, 301, 303, 671-77, 708
 in industrial settings 298
 rural 672
 See also Cardiopulmonary resuscitation; First aid
Health-Illness Profile (H-IP) 669
Health maintenance organizations
 bibliographies on 18, 20
 emergency services education in 308
Heart attacks, bibliography on 29. See also Coronary care units
Helen Hayes Hospital. Spinal Cord Unit (West Haverstraw, N.Y.) 605
Helicopters. See Air transportation
Hennepin County Medical Center (Minneapolis) 538, 713
Hospital emergency services 399, 573, 614
 administration of 19, 267
 bibliographies on 14-15, 18, 19, 23-24, 30
 categorization of 463-500
 community involvement in 638, 644
 as competition for private practitioners 559
 disaster planning in 509-10, 737-40, 742-43, 764, 768, 773-75, 779, 782-84, 786-87
 EMS transportation services of 354, 388, 397, 438, 459
 finance of 467-68, 510, 544, 577
 legal aspects 23, 484, 656
 poison cases and the 607
 psychiatry in 299, 305, 475, 526, 529, 627
 review and evaluation 678-79, 685, 687-88, 691, 693, 700, 707, 711, 716, 723, 727, 732

 rural 489, 495-96, 519, 539-40, 544, 555
 social worker roles in 246
 space and utilization of space 10, 18, 476-77, 501-65, 701
 staffing (plans, needs, problems) 244-45, 248, 260-61, 264-65, 269-70, 273, 281, 283, 289, 293, 299-300, 304, 307, 309, 311, 483, 519, 530, 541, 544
 triage in 283, 307, 508, 521, 523, 537, 551, 558, 564, 678, 743-44
 in university medical centers 471
 See also Intensive care units; Nurses, emergency room; Outpatient services; Patient care; Physicians, in emergency care
Hospital for Joint Diseases and Medical Center (N.Y. City) 633
Hospital for Sick Children. Neonatal Intensive Care Unit (Toronto) 616
Hospital of Charleroi 390
Hospital Reserve Disaster Inventory (HRDI) 757
Houston
 ambulance service in 407
 emergency coronary care in 435
Hungary, paramedical education in 393
Hysteria, emergency treatment of 650

I

Illinois
 ambulance services in 367
 EMS evaluation in 699
 hospital emergency facilities in 472
  utilization studies 512
 trauma patient care system in 578, 603
Illinois, University of. Research Resources Laboratory 652
Illinois Trauma Program 280, 721-22
Indiana
 burn care in 588
 EMS councils in 636
Infants (newborn), care of ill 615-26
 regional programs 615

Subject Index

transportation in 424, 453, 616, 618-20, 622, 624
Information systems and management, bibliographies on 9-10, 20
Institute for Scientific Information p.12
Intensive care units 571, 574, 583, 614
  bibliography on 19
  design of 567, 579
  mobile
    evaluation of 728-29
    for the newborn 453
  nurses in 294-95
  personnel needed for 262
  See also types of ICUs (e.g., Coronary care units)
Intermountain Regional Poison Control Center (Utah) 612
International Rescue and First Aid Association 221
Interns; internships, emergency department training and 304
Interphase EMS Foundation 222
Iowa, hospital emergency services in 478
Ireland
  disaster management in 768
  emergency coronary care in 430

J

Johns Hopkins Hospital (Baltimore) 526
  Adult Emergency Department 732
Johns Hopkins University. School of Medicine 521
Johnson (Robert Wood) Foundation 2, 6, 370
Joint Commission on Accreditation of Hospitals 275, 656, 784

K

Kansas City, Mo., hospital emergency facilities in 485, 500
  utilization studies 536
Kansas City General Hospital and Medical Center 536
Kentucky
  ambulance service in 389
  hospital emergency facilities in 489
King County, Wash., out-of-hospital cardiac arrest studies of 695, 697

L

Little Company of Mary Hospital (Torrance, Calif.) 294
London, Engl., disaster planning in 745
London, Ont., disaster planning in 753
Los Angeles; Los Angeles County
  ambulance service in 334, 384, 395, 408
  disaster planning in 312, 735
  folk medicine beliefs of Mexican-Americans in 548
Los Angeles County-University of Southern California Medical Center 254, 531
Lower classes. See Poor

M

McCullough-Hyde Memorial Hospital (Oxford, Ohio) 269
Madison, Wis.
  EMS transportation system in 352
  neonatal care in 626
Maine
  EMS communication systems in 336
  EMS transportation systems in 342
Malpractice. See Medical law
MarAd Satellite Navigation-Communication System 330
Martha Eliot Health Center (Boston) 522
Maryland, emergency helicopter services in 439
Maryland, University of. Center for Study of Trauma 439
Maryland Emergency Medical Services Communications System 317
Maryland Institute for Emergency Medical Services 445, 570, 581, 763
Maryland Institute for Emergency Medicine 569, 572
Maryland State Intensive Care Neonatal Program (MSICNP) 621-23
Massachusetts, EMS transportation systems in 355
Massachusetts General Hospital 325
Mathematical models. See Models (mathematical and computer)
Medical care. See Patient care

Subject Index

Medical College of Georgia. Burn Treatment Center 594
Medical College of Pennsylvania 666
Medical College of Virginia. Department of Anesthesiology 266
Medical education
  bibliography on 21
  first aid and EMS training in 247, 266, 277, 288
  See also types of people educated (e.g., Nurses; Physicians)
Medical equipment, bibliography on 16
  cost effectiveness 13
  See also Ambulance services, equipment and design
Medical law
  emergency room 484, 656
  bibliography on 23
  the emergency medical technician and 243
  state, as a barrier to EMS development 712
Medical personnel, bibliographies on 19, 21. See also Emergency medical technicians and paramedics; Nurses; Physicians
Medical records. See Patient care, record keeping in
Medical social workers
  in emergency department care 246
  in intensive unit care 262
Medicare, impact on Quebec hospital utilization 552
Memorial Hospital (Anaheim, Calif.) 574
Memphis, Tenn., EMS evaluation in 706
Menominie, Wis., ambulance service in 388
Mexican Americans, medical folk beliefs of. See also Spanish-speaking Americans
Miami, emergency coronary care in 430
Michigan, University of. Hospital. Burn Center 587
Mid-Anglia General Practitioner Accident Service 358
Mid-Coast Comprehensive Health Planning Association 350
Middlesex Memorial Hospital (Connecticut) 543
Military, assistance to EMS by 446, 458, 460

bibliography on 17
in California 350, 455
training for 282
Mississippi
  emergency helicopter services in 451
  hospital emergency facility utilization in 539
Missouri, EMS communication systems in 340
Models (mathematical and computer)
  bibliography on 17
  for burn care 590
  in disaster planning 785
  of EMS assessment 689, 701, 709, 711
  of EMS councils 639
  of EMS transportation systems 346, 352-53, 363, 374, 378-79, 382-84, 395, 404, 407-8, 410, 444, 494, 719, 730
  of hospital categorization 487, 498-99
  of hospital utilization 516, 518, 525, 534, 545, 554
  of rural health education 672
  of the severity of patient illnesses 658
Montreal, hospital emergency facility utilization in 552
Morrisania City Hospital (Bronx) 528
Mount Zion Hospital (San Francisco) 337

N

National Academy of Sciences 297
  Committee on Emergency Rooms 500
  See also National Research Council-National Academy of Sciences
National Association of Emergency Medical Technicians 223
National Association of Emergency Paramedics 224
National Audio-Visual Center 199
National Burn Information Exchange 596
National Clearinghouse for Emergency Medical Services 7, p. 12
National Emergency Medical Services Information Clearinghouse (NEMSIC) 8

Subject Index

National Highway Safety Act (1966) p. 2, 1, 690
National League of Nursing 778
National Library of Medicine p. 12
National Poison Center Network 610
National Registry of Emergency Medical Technicians 225
National Research Council-National Academy of Sciences 491
 Division of Medical Sciences. Committees on Trauma and Shock 236
National Safety Council 361
National Spinal Injuries Centre (Geneva) 602
National Technical Information Service p. 12
Nebraska, EMS communication systems in 332, 340
Neighborhood health centers. See Health centers, neighborhood
Netherlands, emergency coronary care in 426
New Hampshire, emergency-outpatient satellite facilities in 544
New Haven, Conn.
 hospital emergency facility utilization in 507
 rape counseling in 628
New Jersey, EMS communication systems in 340
New River Valley Planning District Emergency Medical Service Communications System 338
New York City
 ambulance service in 385
 disaster planning in 755-56
 emergency coronary care in 430
New York State
 burn care in 590
 hospital emergency facility utilization in 503-4, 519
New Zealand, prehospital trauma care in 343
North Carolina
 emergency helicopter services in 454
 EMS evaluation in 726
North Memorial Medical Center (Minneapolis) 713
Norway, ambulance services in 396
Nuclear war, planning for 772
 bibliography on 29
 See also Fallout shelters

Nurses, emergency care 256, 289-91, 311, 687
 acceptance of 241
 in burn care 591
 in disaster planning 764, 778
 education of 248, 260, 300, 475
  bibliography on 23
  rural areas 309
 evaluation of 911 calls by 385
 in intensive care units 294-95, 566
 in neonatal care 623
 the psychiatric nurse 305
 triage by 283, 307, 521, 678

O

O'Hare Airport (Chicago) disaster planning at 761
Ohio
 EMS evaluation in 699, 708
 EMS transportation services in 345
 health education in 673
 hospital emergency services in 491, 497
Oklahoma
 ambulance services in rural 375
 hospital emergency facility utilization in 555
Oklahoma City, Okla., hospital emergency facility utilization in 560
Oswego County, N.Y., hospital emergency facility utilization in 504
Outpatient services 503, 506, 527, 542, 544, 550, 614
 bibliographies on 19-20

P

Packaged Disaster Hospital (PDH) program 757, 773-75, 783
Paramedics. See Emergency medical technicians and paramedics
Patient care (accessibility, delivery, etc.) 645-46
 advocacy programs in 732
 bibliographies on 10, 20-21, 23-24
 record keeping in 647-70, 727
 See also subheadings "space and utilization of spaces" and "review and evaluation" under Hospitals, emergency services

Subject Index

Pediatrics
  emergency care in 548, 565
  triage in 564
  See also Infants (newborn)
Pennsylvania
  burn care in 586, 593
  emergency coronary care in 422
  spinal cord injury care in 601
  trauma victim care system in 576
Pennsylvania, University of. Center for the Study of Emergency Health Services 258, 272, 292. See also National Emergency Medical Services Information Clearinghouse
Pennsylvania, University of. Graduate Hospital. Emergency Service Community Advisory Board 638
Philadelphia, EMS communication system in 314
Physicians
  in emergency care 242, 259, 264, 281
    acceptance of emergency nurse practitioners by 241
    as ambulance attendants 390, 396
    in disaster management 736
    education and training of 244-45, 252, 303, 304
      bibliography on 23
      CPR skills 731
    in EMT ambulance training 310
    foreign born 270
    planning and control roles of p. 2, 279, 512
    recruitment for rural areas 544
  in private practice 559
    primary group practice 557
  See also Interns; Residents
Physicians assistants 300
  education and training of 255, 261
Pittsburgh Poison Center 610
Poisoning 606-12
Police
  EMS interaction with 353
  EMS transportation services of 354-55
Pontiac Plan 264-65
Poor, demand for medical care by 645
Presbyterian Hospital (New York City) 518
Problem-Oriented Medical Record (POMR) 647-48, 660, 663
Psychiatry, in emergency medicine 299, 305, 414, 475, 526, 529, 627
Public safety agencies. See Fire departments; Police
Public Safety Officers Foundation 235, 643

R

Rape
  counseling 628
  of males 631
Regional Pediatric Trauma Center (Chicago, Ill.) 603
Rehabilitation, bibliography on 21
Rehabilitation Act (1973) 601
Residents; residencies, in emergency medicine 244-45, 265, 274-75, 293, 304
  psychiatric training for 299
Respiratory therapists 262
Resuscitation 538
  equipment for 341, 704. See also Cardiopulmonary resuscitation
Rochester, N.Y., hospital emergency facility utilization in 527, 553
Royal Victoria Hospital (Belfast) 768
Rural areas
  EMS for 285
  ambulance services 375, 386, 397-98, 401, 417, 419
  bibliographies on 14, 16, 20-22, 31
    transportation services 17
  burn care in 595
  coronary care in 422, 428
  emergency helicopter services in 443, 448
  emergency nurse training in 309
  hospital services in 489, 495-96, 519
    utilization studies 539-40, 544, 555
  volunteer services in 353
  health education in 672
Russia
  emergency coronary care in 430
  emergency psychiatric services in 414

S

Sacramento, disaster planning in 749

Subject Index

St. Louis Hospital 273
St. Louis University. Hospital 459
St. Mary's Hospital (Waterbury, Conn.) 517
St. Vincent's Hospital (New York City) 430
Salem County, N.J., disaster planning in 741
San Berbadino, Calif., geographic pattern of EMS demand in 359
San Diego, University of. Hospital. Regional Trauma Center 566
San Francisco, EMS communication system in 313
San Francisco General Hospital 283
Seattle, EMS transportation system in 349
Ships, emergency medical communications for 330
Shreveport, La., EMS communication system in 333
Snowmobiles, as EMS vehicles 354
Social workers. See Medical social workers
Society for Critical Care Medicine 226
Society for Total Emergency Programs (STEP) 228
Society of Teachers of Emergency Medicine 227
South Africa, emergency mobile accident units in 427
South Carolina, emergency helicopter services in 446
South Community Hospital (Oklahoma City) 560
Southeast Ohio. Emergency Medical Services Demonstration Project 708
Southern California, University of. School of Medicine. Department of Emergency Medicine 727
Spanish-speaking Americans, EMS utilization by 515
  information services for 674
  See also Mexican-Americans
Spinal cord injury 600–605
  regional programs for treating 600
Sporting events, disaster planning for 765, 767
State government, emergency medical support by 4, 712

for ambulance services 376
Strokes, bibliography on 29
Suicide 607, 609, 630
Switzerland
  neonatal care in 624
  spinal cord injury care in 602
Syracuse, N.Y., hospital emergency facility utilization in 504
System Input Severity Measure 705

T

Telecommunication. See Communications
Television in medicine. See Communications
Texas, ambulance services in 412
Tompkins County (N.Y.) Hospital 504
Traffic accidents
  bibliography on injuries resulting from 29
  communications in emergency medical services for 326
  helicopter ambulances in servicing 444–45, 451
  study of emergency care in 692
  trauma care following 578
Traffic safety, bibliographies on 19, 32
Transportation services 341–462, 464
  automatic vehicle location systems 346
  bibliographies on 9, 16–17, 24
  in burn care 589
  guidelines and standards 354
  in neonatal care 424, 453, 616, 618–20, 622, 624
  See also types of transportation services (e.g., Ambulance services; Coronary care units, mobile)
Trauma care 566–84, 603
  administration and coordination of programs for 280, 582
  bibliography on 9
  communications in 326
  computerized registries in 652
  emergency nursing in 291
  evaluation of 708
  financial aspects 577
  hospital services for 472, 475
  prehospital emergency care and transportation in 343, 351
  regional centers for 566, 568

Subject Index

trauma indexes 763
Triage systems. See Disaster planning and management, triage in; Hospital emergency services, triage in
Tulare, Calif., ambulance service in 397
Tulsa, Okla., EMS communication system in 319

U

United Kingdom
  disaster management in 768
  emergency helicopter services in 452
  EMS evaluation in 692
  trauma patient care in 584
  prehospital 343
  See also Ireland; London, Engl.
U.S. Army. Medical Unit Self-Contained Transportable Hospital 511. See also Military
U.S. Department of Health and Human Services. Division of Emergency Medical Services 239, 275
U.S. Department of Health, Education and Welfare 494, 702
  Division of Emergency Medical Service 699
  National Center for Health Services Research 521
U.S. Department of Transportation 250, 450
  Basic Training Program for Emergency Medical Technicians-Ambulance 329
  National Highway Traffic Safety Administration. Rescue and Emergency Medical Services Division 240
U.S. Federal Aviation Agency 461
U.S. Federal Communications Commission 236, 313, 328
U.S. Fire Service 634

U.S. Office of Telecommunication Policy 238
University Association for EMS 229
Urban areas, EMS for
  ambulance services 392, 407, 413
  bibliographies on 14, 20
  education and training 287
  transportation services 17
  hospital utilization studies of 535
Utah, poison control centers in 612

V

Vermont
  ambulance services in 418
  hospital emergency facilities in 496
  utilization studies 530
Virginia
  burn care in 589
  emergency coronary care in 421, 428
  standardized ambulance reporting form of 670
Virginia, University of
  School of Medicine 247
  School of Nursing 260

W

Washtenaw County, Mich., ambulance service in 417
Western Pennsylvania Regional Medical Program 364
West Virginia
  ambulance services in 401
  emergency coronary care in 423
  emergency helicopter services in 443, 448
Wisconsin
  ambulance service in 398
  EMS communication systems in 340
  EMS councils in 682
  hospital emergency facilities in 463
    utilization studies 501
  neonatal care in 615, 617